The
Mindful
Social
Worker

Living your best
social work life

Other books you may be interested in:

Safeguarding Adults Together under the Care Act 2014: A Multi-agency Practice Guide
Barbara Starns   978-1-913063-25-2

Social Exclusion in the UK: The Lived Experience
Edited by Mel Hughes   978-1-914171-86-4

Young Refugees and Asylum Seekers: The Truth About Britain
Declan Henry   978-1-913063-97-9

Dilemmas and Decision Making in Social Work
Abbi Jackson   978-1-914171-20-8

Social Work and Covid-19: Lessons for Education and Practice
Edited by Denise Turner   978-1-913453-61-9

Out of the Shadows: The Role of Social Workers in Disasters
Edited by Angie Bartoli, Maris Stratulis
and Rebekah Pierre   978-1-915080-07-3

The Anti-racist Social Worker: Stories of Activism by Social Care and Allied Health Professionals
Edited by Tanya Moore and Glory Simango   978-1-914171-41-3

To order, or for details of our bulk discounts, please go to our website www.criticalpublishing.com or contact our distributor, Ingram Publisher Services (IPS UK), 10 Thornbury Road, Plymouth PL6 7PP, telephone 01752 202301 or email IPSUK.orders@ingramcontent.com.

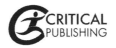

The
Mindful
Social
Worker

Living your best
social work life

BARBARA STARNS

First published in 2022 by Critical Publishing Ltd

British Library Cataloguing in Publication Data
A CIP record for this book is available from the British Library

ISBN: 978-1-915080-35-6

This book is also available in the following e-book formats:
EPUB ISBN: 978-1-915080-36-3
Adobe e-book ISBN: 978-1-915080-37-0
Audio book ISBN: 978-1-915080-99-8

Cover and text design by Out of House Limited
Project Management by Newgen Publishing UK
Printed and bound in Great Britain by 4edge, Essex

Critical Publishing
3 Connaught Road
St Albans
AL3 5RX

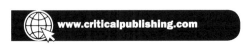

Printed on FSC accredited paper

Contents

Drink your tea slowly and reverently, as it if is the axis on which the world earth revolves slowly, evenly, without rushing toward the future

Thich Nhat Hanh

Acknowledgements

Thanks as always to Jon and Ollie B for support, patience and lots of tea, as well as to Di at Critical Publishing.

Thanks also to Presenter Media for the desk-swipe template.

About the author

Barbara Starns has worked as a social worker and social work manager for nearly 30 years, in both children's and adult services. She currently works as an author, independent consultant and specialist trainer. Barbara has a lifelong practice of meditation and yoga. She has devised and is delivering mindfulness meditation courses for staff at Hull City Council and is undertaking her professional teaching qualifications in mindful meditation with Sarah Presley at the British School of Meditation.

Introduction

Mindfulness, the practice of presence in the moment with an attitude of openness and acceptance, has become a feature of modern living. It has expanded from its religious origins to become a wider secular concept that incorporates a wide variety of definitions and techniques. Perhaps the most prevalent of these in the Western world has been the concept of mindfulness propagated by Jon Kabat-Zinn in the 1970s.

Paying attention in a particular way: on purpose, in the present moment, and non-judgementally.

(Kabat-Zinn, 1994, p 4)

Whatever version of mindfulness is adopted, it is certain that mindful practice is gaining traction within personal, professional and policy areas of life (Brown et al, 2015) as a means of harnessing the positive benefits identified by research into the subject. Social work is no exception, as the shared values of compassion, respect, kindness and open-mindedness make mindfulness a natural ally of the caring professions. Initially embraced to support social work self-care and mitigate stress-related pressure in the workplace, attention is now being given to the application of mindfulness to social work practice, with the prospect of ensuing positive outcomes for people who use social services (Trowbridge and Mische-Lawson, 2016). While research into the impact of mindfulness on the social work profession is at its embryonic stage, many studies demonstrate the value of mindful practice in this area. Notably, the positive effects include: improved management of emotions, enhanced thinking and decision-making skills, the potential for stronger interpersonal relationships and greater ability to reduce judgemental bias (McGarrigle and Walsh, 2011; Wong, 2013; Kinman et al, 2020; McCusker, 2020). The resulting legitimisation of mindfulness on the mainstream stage of health and social care prompts broader consideration of this topic, requiring we look at ways that it can strengthen social work intervention in support of the vulnerable while also promoting the well-being of professionals themselves (MAPPG, 2015).

This book takes the reader on a unique, mindful practice journey to explore how mindfulness can not only provide a means of improving care for the self as a social worker but can also extend into practice to increase the efficacy of social work as well. It builds on established research, professional information and guidance about the relationship between mindfulness and the social work role, with practice tools, case study reflections and self-assessments to enable any practitioner, from newly qualified students to experienced social workers or caring professionals, to incorporate mindfulness into their practical working lives to positive effect. It does so within the framework of professional standards for social work education and practice, demonstrating the ease with which mindfulness relates to the architecture of the social work profession.

Above all else, at times of difficulty, within a job that presents many challenges, this book is about kindness, compassion, joy and taking care of self while also caring for others.

References and further reading

Beres, L (2009) Mindfulness and Reflexitivity: The No-Self as Reflexive Practitioner. In Hick, S F (ed) *Mindfulness and Social Work*. Chicago: Lyceum Books.

Brown, K W, Creswell, J D and Ryan, M (2015) Introduction: The Evolution of Mindfulness Science. In Brown, K W, Creswell, J D and Ryan, M (eds) *Handbook of Mindfulness* (pp 1–6). New York: Guildford Publications.

Kabat-Zinn, J (1994) *Wherever You Go, There You Are: Mindfulness Meditation in Everyday Life*. New York: Hachette.

Kinman, K, Grant, L and Kelly, S (2020) 'It's My Secret Space': The Benefits of Mindfulness for Social Workers. *The British Journal of Social Work*, 50(3): 758–77.

McCusker, P (2020) Mindfulness in Social Work Education and Practice. Insight 56. *Iriss*. [online] Available at: www.iriss.org.uk/resources/insig hts/mindfulness-social-work-education-and-practice#:~:text=Mindfuln ess%20can%20help%20increase%20awareness,enhancing%20think ing%20and%20interpersonal%20skills (accessed 18 August 2022).

McGarrigle, T and Walsh, C A (2011) Mindfulness, Self-Care, and Wellness in Social Work: Effects of Contemplative Training. *Journal of Religion & Spirituality in Social Work: Social Thought*, 30(3): 212–33.

Mindfulness All-Party Parliamentary Group (2015) *Mindful Nation UK*. [online] Available at: www.themindfulnessinitiative.org/Handlers/Downl oad.ashx?IDMF=1af56392-4cf1-4550-bdd1-72e809fa627a (accessed 18 August 2022).

Rajan-Rankin, S (2014) Self-Identity, Embodiment and the Development of Emotional Resilience. *British Journal of Social Work*, 44(8): 2426–42.

Trowbridge, K and Mische Lawson, L (2016) Mindfulness-Based Interventions with Social Workers and the Potential for Enhanced Patient-Centred Care: A Systematic Review of the Literature. *Social Work in Health Care*, 55(2): 101–24.

Turner, K (2009) Mindfulness: The Present Moment in Clinical Social Work. *Clinical Social Work Journal*, 37(2): 95–103.

Wong, Y-L-R (2013) Returning to Silence, Connecting to Wholeness: Contemplative Pedagogy for Critical Social Work Education. *Journal of Religion & Spirituality in Social Work: Social Thought*, 32(3): 269–85.

Chapter 1

Mindfulness and social work

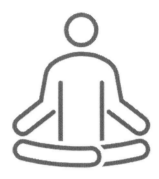

Mindfulness is meditation in action, dependent on a 'be here now' approach.

(Borysenko, 1987)

As the term 'mindfulness' becomes more common within our modern world, it is both interesting and possibly frustrating for scientific measurement that there remains an absence of consensus about what the term means, that the world still lacks an agreed definition of the concept. But the truth of the matter seems to be that mindfulness is a non-verbal, experiential activity that cannot be reduced to a short definition; it seems to have different meanings for different people, manifesting in a variety of forms. It is a subject that requires acceptance that agreement might be reached about some features and characteristics of mindfulness, but a consensus on what it is may not be achieved in the short term. This chapter will explore not only the signature of mindfulness, how to access the mindful state and how mindfulness manifests itself, but also its compatibility with social work, an occupation that naturally lends itself to the incorporation of mindfulness to positive effect.

A significant body of research and academic discourse has developed over several years, identifying mindfulness as an obvious adjunct tool to the social work role that adds value to practice and ensuing outcomes for people who receive social work support. This chapter will shine a light on that relationship to enable the reader to reflect and consider for themselves if mindfulness might play a part in their professional lives, and if so in what way. Ultimately the decision to become a mindful social worker lies with the professional, but here consideration can be given to the argument for the adoption of a mindful approach, one that is gaining traction in social work as in many other professional worlds.

This chapter will include:

Defining the impossible: mindfulness

Historical context

Features of a mindful mind

Becoming mindful

The benefits of mindfulness

A balanced approach

The mindful social work partnership

Defining the impossible: mindfulness

Mindfulness is most commonly described as the art of showing up in the here and now, and doing so with open acceptance of the moment as it unfolds. A small, simple act that encompasses so much that is beneficial, predominantly the development of a calm, wise and considered approach to life: *'Paying attention in a particular way: on purpose, in the present moment, and non-judgmentally'* (Kabat-Zinn, 1994). Observing the present, without judgement, enables full awareness of actuality to emerge, rather than a fabricated interpretation of reality dominated by a personal perspective. Presence for the experience, whether good or bad, creates space for the generation of greater insight into the emotional reactions, physical sensations and habitual responses to situations (Teasdale and Chaskalson, 2011). In turn, the practice provides opportunities for wise, considered action rather than repetitive automation based on the learned behaviour of the past or worries about the future; the latter described in Buddhist terms as sleepwalking through life.

Eventually the mindful person can develop a sense of detachment from moments, broadening their vision of what is taking place, awakening a form of attention that extends beyond insight into external events as they unfold, to include observation of the self in response to events, most usually referred to as 'watcher' or 'seer' abilities. This enables a more objective understanding of what is happening, with increased control over the mind, enhancing the ability of self to make connections between thoughts, beliefs, and actions. *'Gradually we can train ourselves to notice when our thoughts are taking over and realise that thoughts are simple "mental events" that do not have to control us'* (Williams, 2018). Awareness affords us the ability to act wisely rather than respond quickly in ways that are sometimes later viewed with regret or which perpetuate the bad habits that often warrant change.

Take home message

Mindfulness is the simple practice of living in the present, often difficult to achieve, but offering the prospect of positive personal growth through perseverance.

Historical context

Mindfulness, and in particular its meditative form, has been hiding in plain sight for centuries; rooted in ancient religious tradition, it is documented in religious tracts available for historical reference. Although it is most closely associated with Buddhism, Hinduism has an extensive record of mindful practice predating that of Buddhism. However, unsurprisingly, given the ability of mindfulness to silence the mind, it has been present throughout history in many religions, including Islam, Christianity and Judaism, to name but a few. The practice is viewed as essential to the pursuit of spiritual enlightenment beyond the cares of daily life (Trousselard et al, 2014; Ridgeon, 2003).

The transition of mindfulness from the religious pursuit of spiritual enlightenment to the secular practice familiar today in the modern Western world is believed to have begun around the 1950s with the expansion of travel affording more people contact with Eastern philosophy and meditation. The transition of Eastern spiritual practice increased in momentum in the 1970s when mindfulness began to be used as an experimental treatment for psychological conditions. Perhaps the most noteworthy of these innovations was the mindfulness-based stress reduction programme of therapy initiated by among others Jon Kabat-Zinn. The ensuing success of the programme gave credibility to mindfulness as a viable treatment for mental health (Logan, 2014), encouraging others to consider where else mindfulness might be of help in the world of psychological intervention.

Anecdotal reports that positive outcomes could be achieved through the application of mindfulness to specific psychological conditions prompted scientific interest and research to find out what, if any, the benefits might be to the human condition. The results have catapulted mindfulness to front and centre stage. Academic institutions devote specialised departments to its study; government policy documents advocate the application of mind-fulness to emerging health and well-being challenges; and institutions adopt mindful approaches to garner positive change for individuals and communities (for example, the Oxford University Mindfulness Centre, the Bangor University Centre for Mindfulness Research and Practice and the Mindfulness All-Party Parliamentary Group UK (MAPPG)). A blossoming research community has grown around the subject exploring what, on the face of it, appears to be limitless opportunities for application.

However, mindfulness's rapid expansion into the mainstream has prompted notes of caution from many observers concerned about an over-reliance on mindfulness as a panacea for all problems, particularly where it has been used to place responsibility for good health and well-being solely with the individual, diluting the duties of care that lie with governments and organisations. The term 'McMindfulness' (Purser, 2019) has also been coined to highlight the overuse of the concept for commer-cial exploitation. The debate is a useful one, and while not suggesting the abandonment of a practice that has proven benefits, it does highlight the need for individuals to research the subject for themselves, exercising judgement over the wealth of literature that is now available for use.

Take home message

Mindfulness has an ancient heritage that establishes the authenticity of the practice itself, identifying it as a pursuit worthy of consideration in the social work context. But the term is so widely used in all aspects of our lives that careful consideration should be given to the provenance of the mindful material available.

Features of a mindful mind

 There is general agreement among those studying the effects of mindfulness that it can develop a calmer, more peaceful mind, alongside the possibility of reduced if not eliminated internal chatter (Carmody and Baer, 2008; Lazar et al, 2005). In contrast with the experience of mindless reactivity, mindfulness is seen as a method to achieve a more measured, centred response to the present. Gradually, as the detached observation of the self becomes dominant, a perceptual shift takes place in the degree of awareness and control a person gain (Carmody and Baer, 2008), replacing habitual reactivity with wise, intuitive responses. Mindful practice, through open acceptance without judgement, cultivates kindness and compassion towards the self and others, qualities that enhance human relationships as well as individual well-being (Lazar et al, 2005). The resultant reduction in critical thoughts is believed to lead to a more confident, contented mind, less encumbered by anxious or fearful feelings. Over-reliance on past experiences to negotiate the present is reduced through mindfulness, minimising the prospect of repeating the same mistakes, ones that we would intentionally like to avoid. It is felt that a mindful mind becomes a new mind, open to every experience, with a new perspective, unencumbered by the application of old thought patterns that might blindfold us to new possibilities or choices.

Mindful point of reflection

Bring to mind a time when you have had to respond to an emergency or life-changing event when the news has been unexpected. Try to remember how your mind responded: Did it seem like the world slowed down? Did it feel you had more time and space to react? Were other distractions blocked out by your focus or concentration?

This experience is similar to the reported changes that meditation practitioners report in their everyday lives to a varying degree.

Becoming mindful

 While recent years have seen growth in the popularity of mindfulness, with a commercial industry offering services to support mindful activity, it should be remembered that mindfulness is free. It is a quality or ability that exists within us all. Just like the fight or flight response evolved to help deal with danger, humans also have the skill of letting go of inner chatter, reducing reactivity and paying attention to a moment as it presents itself without judgement or expectation. However, it is a quality that needs to be recognised and nurtured; the ability exists within everyone, but it is only through self-determination that mindfulness can be brought to the forefront of one's life.

Many people naturally tune into their mindful abilities and are able to access a mindful state with ease, but for others there is a need to undertake activities that lead them to arrive at a mindful state. Meditation is viewed as the form of practice that most effectively generates mindfulness, sitting quietly with eyes closed, focusing on the breath as it enters and leaves the body. While meditation is a simple task, it is often not simple to practise. Frequently, when sitting quietly, focusing on the breath, inner chatter and thoughts seem to increase. This chatter is always present but comes to the fore when the opportunity to sit quietly is taken.

One of the key elements of meditation practice is therefore learning to let go, to observe the chatter without reaction or judgement. Starved of attention, after much practice the chatter subsides, allowing the meditator to move towards a quieter, calmer state of mind. It is this practice that affects all aspects of the meditator's life, resulting in the positive benefits now observed by scientific research. Initial meditation practice can be uncomfortable for the meditator, as it can be difficult to sit quietly, focused on breath, with the invasion of many thoughts, some of which might be unwelcome. The commitment to practise regularly allows the meditator to develop the ability to be present to difficult experiences and to notice how the mind works by observing thought in a detached fashion. The art of waiting for our inner dialogue to subside also teaches the skill of creating space around thought or action in daily life. Resources to help support a mindfulness practice are available at the end of this book in the Resource hut.

The benefits of mindfulness

Research studies have demonstrated mindful practice can reduce anxiety, combat depression and balance emotions (Davidson et al, 2003; Erisman and Roemer, 2010; Farb et al, 2010; Hoffman et al, 2010). But research also indicates that the benefits of mindfulness can extend beyond mental well-being, to the daily long-term functioning of the mind, serving to reduce our reactivity (Ortner et al, 2007; Cahn and Polich, 2009) and enabling a more considered approach to problem-solving. This approach incorporates creative thought to find solutions, while also offering advantages for the development of capacities for compassion and empathy, core components of good social work practice.

The science bit

 Notwithstanding its presence in religion for many centuries, mindfulness is currently being studied like never before, the difference being that it has drawn intensive scientific attention as evidence emerges that mindfulness can change the physical nature of the brain. In short, the effects of mindfulness can be evidenced in brain and body physicality. New discoveries about how the brain works have been a game changer for this burgeoning area of scientific research; in essence, something called neuroplasticity has entered the neuroscience field, and this has changed the way the community views brain development.

Neuroplasticity

Traditionally, the brain had been viewed as a finite organ that develops through childhood, reaching optimum functionality in early adulthood before decline during old age. But technological advances have disproved this belief through the detection of a phenomenon known as neuroplasticity. This newly discovered feature of the brain demonstrates that it grows and shrinks dependent on the demands made upon it rather than because of age and stage of life. The brain can grow neural connections to master new tasks and discard old ones that are not needed, all the while maintaining connections that carry out everyday functions. The brain is both adaptable and responsive to change, and the changes can be scientifically measured. This discovery has proved important for mindfulness research because it has meant that scientists have finally been able to observe the impact mindful meditation makes in quantifiable terms. Evidence has been emerging that the brain can be trained and retrained at any age. Mindfulness studies subsequent to this discovery have shown that new ways of approaching the mind can result in long-term changes for the development of the brain (Wolkin, 2015).

We know that people who consistently meditate have a singular ability to cultivate positive emotions, retain emotional stability, and engage in mindful behaviour. The observed differences in brain anatomy might give us a clue why meditators have these exceptional abilities.

(*Science Daily*, 2009)

Good to know changes in the brain

 Research studies thus far have noted observable changes in several areas of brain development, scientifically verifiable through measurement and scans, that are the result of mindful meditation. Growth in the grey matter of the anterior cingulate cortex has been noted among those who have a meditation practice. Expansion of this region of the brain is linked to enhanced executive functions associated with self-regulation, the ability to respond to conflicting demands for attention, more commonly known as multitasking, and greater cognitive flexibility (Lazar et al, 2005).

Mindfulness meditation also increases cortical thickness in the hippocampus element of the limbic system, the area of the brain that governs learning and memory, which is also susceptible to stress. Growth in cortical thickness is believed to result in stress relief (Carmody, 2009).

Conversely, mindfulness appears to result in decreases in the amygdala, which is responsible for the fight or flight response needed for survival, something which in the modern world often cannot be switched off when no longer needed, resulting in increased anxiety and fear. Regular mindful practice reduces cell volume in this area, alleviating those unwanted feelings (Holzel et al, 2010).

In addition, closer study has been given to the effects of mindfulness on the default mode network of the brain. This network is often linked to wandering thoughts or the concept of our 'inner chimp', which refers to a directionless movement from thought to thought without connection or intent. Carmody (2009) felt that the resultant rumination activity contributes to an unhappiness that can result in depression. A study completed by Judson et al in 2011 found a deactivation of the default mode network among experienced meditators, suggesting meditation as a means of reducing the effects of the default mode, logically leading to a calmer, more contented mind. An additional study by Carmody and Baer in 2008 reinforces Judson et al's conclusions, highlighting the discovery that mindfulness counteracts tendencies of rumination, leading to an improved sense of happiness and well-being among practitioners. Participants in these studies confirmed these positive changes in mood in anecdotal reporting, information that correlates with the observation of changes in brain function. Findings also included stronger neural connections in the areas of the brain associated with cognition and self-management.

The positive effects of mindfulness are not only detectable in the grey matter of the brain, they are also visible in our whole-body reactions. Indeed Kabat-Zinn (1990) reports that the benefits observed through the mindful-based stress reduction programme were initially mainly physical rather than mind orientated. As early as 1975, Benson et al conducted a study into the physical reactions of the body to meditation. They observed a link between meditation and lower rates of oxygen consumption and blood pressure, labelling them as the relaxation response. Further research into these reactions have found the relaxation response is effective in the treatment of high blood pressure, reducing the need for medication (Dusek et al, 2008). Scientific research has also found that mindful meditation can improve immune functioning within the body. Davison et al (2003) conducted a randomised controlled study into the effects of mindful meditation within a work environment of healthy employees. The study identified not only positive changes in the brain but an increased presence of antibodies indicative of improved immune response capabilities. Participants confirmed improved feelings of wellness, with increased feelings of positive emotions leading to greater happiness. Finally, research carried out by Epel et al in 2009 suggests mindfulness could play a part in slowing the rate of cellular aging. Epel et al highlight the importance of telomeres – strips of atoms on the end of chromosomes – that provide protection from age-related diseases. While stress reduces the length of telomeres, Epel et al have found that mindful meditation has a part to play in promoting and maintaining telomeres, protecting them from the damage of stress and supporting their continued effectiveness.

Mindful point of reflection

The scientific information is a great deal to take in, particularly as it is such a lively research area currently. It might help at this point to take a moment to reflect on the information and consider if you would like to do your own further exploration. Resources are provided in the Resource hut at the end of this book to get you started.

A balanced approach

 Despite the scientific confirmation of mindful benefits, it would be unwise to view it as a catch-all remedy for all problems. Its legitimacy and effectiveness in particular areas of life are supported by science, but as with all things, a balanced approach is advisable. Research has gathered pace, leading to wider trials with verifiable results in this subject area. But there remain notes of caution about the size and design of some studies.

It is also important to be aware that the application of mindfulness in certain situations can lead to negative as well as positive effects. A particular study of the use of the mindfulness app Calm among students in Scotland found both responses. While most participants reported a positive experience, a small minority did have negative outcomes.

This outcome resonates with other studies in the use of mindfulness, including that of Britton (2019), who examined whether mindfulness can be too much of a good thing. One of the conclusions being: '[*Mindfulness processes*] *are usually beneficial but under certain conditions, for certain people, or at certain levels, their effects can turn negative, have costs or have undesirable effects*'.

Take-home message

Mindfulness has been identified with many benefits and is scientifically proven to help develop insight, kindness, cognitive abilities and emotional regulation. But judicious use of the concept is important, together with an understanding that, as with many things in life, there is no one-size-fits-all approach.

The mindful social work partnership

It can be said that the primary role of social work is to support, protect and empower children, adults, families and communities to achieve well-being, including safety from harm and abuse, and to tackle social injustice and promote inclusion to enable people to achieve the outcomes that matter to them in life.

> *The mission of social work is to enhance the effective functioning and well-being of individuals, families and communities.*
>
> (Logan et al, 2014)

Social workers are guided in this role by professional frameworks, ethical standards and academic research leading to theories of intervention, but successful application of these depends upon the individual approach adopted by the social work practitioner. It is for this reason that a great deal of attention is paid to the professional values, qualities and skills necessary to carry out the role. These include the ability to use compassion and kindness to build trusted relationships with those who engage with services, together with emotional intelligence for self-regulation, alongside the capacity to support others. Assessment and analytical skills also play a key part in making sure that each person receives the right kind of support when it is needed, support that is targeted at clear outcomes. A sense of personhood that reinforces the authority of the social work position is also needed in order to work within service user and co-professional relationships. By its very nature, social work is a collaborative exercise, requiring strong communication skills in order to engage with other professionals and people who need services and to negotiate pathways of intervention that meet holistic needs that both include and extend beyond the presenting problems to enhance well-being. Social work, in essence, is a human activity that requires the practitioner to use self in the promotion of equality and change. This requirement necessitates self-knowledge drawn from critical reflection on both personal and professional actions, alongside those of others, to learn from interactions about what works well and what might also be harmful. The use of self also leads on to the issue of self-care in what can be a demanding, emotionally complex and stressful role. Often identified as the missing social work professional competency, care of self is vitally important both personally and for the care of others.

The positive gains to be found in mindfulness make it an obvious yet perhaps under-recognised adjunct tool for social work. Its acknowledged role in the reduction of stress, resulting in a calmer, more peaceful mind, makes it an ideal method to generate a sense of well-being within a profession that has been identified as one of the most physically and emotionally demanding careers available. The caring professions are increasingly recognising the contribution mindfulness can make to good mental health within this challenging working environment. Embraced by the health service, it has been slow to impact social service workers, but a realisation of its assets is now taking hold.

Beyond self-care, mindfulness also has significant potential to add value to social work efficacy, cementing its position as a natural ally for the profession. The values of mindfulness resonate with the professional standards, ethics and values of social work practice (illustrated in Table 1.1). The open-minded, non-judgemental characteristics enhanced by mindful practice support the maintenance of the value base required to uphold the ethical requirements of the role. The growth of mindful traits such as sensitivity, wise curiosity and compassion serve to enhance the success of considered, proportionate social work intervention in partnership with those who need help. While the ability of mindful practice to develop the characteristics of intelligent enquiry, self-knowledge and considered awareness within the practitioner highlight the essential contribution mindfulness can make to strong communication, growth in learning through critical reflection and the ability to construct and maintain collaborative, trusted relationships are at the heart of transformative social work.

Table 1.1

Social work standards and values	Mindfulness qualities developed through practice
Valuing each person as an individual, recognising their strengths and abilities Respecting human rights, views and wishes Recognising differences across diverse communities	Presence in the moment and non-judgemental acceptance. Improved engagement with individuals, often resulting in greater creativity and enhanced problem-solving. Meeting people where they are not where you think they are.

$\longrightarrow$

Table 1.1 (cont)

Social work standards and values	Mindfulness qualities developed through practice
Recognising and using responsibly the power and authority linked to the social work role	Self-insight, reflection and awareness.
Being open, honest, reliable and fair	Open-mindedness that cultivates new learning, with unbiased curiosity.
Using supervision/feedback to critically reflect and identify learning needs	Considered actions rather than reactivity based on past experience.
Reflecting on own values and challenging their impact in practice	
Recognising where there may be bias in decision-making and addressing issues that might arise from ethical concerns	
Promoting social justice, equality and inclusion	
Respecting and maintaining people's dignity	Openness and acceptance
Practising ways that demonstrate empathy	Increased empathy and compassion
Actively listening to understand people	Presence in the moment and awareness
Treating information about people with sensitivity	Awareness, focus and compassion
Holding different explanations in mind and using evidence to inform decisions	Non-judgemental presence, natural curiosity, improved decision-making

The affinity between mindfulness and social work has itself become the subject of academic research, and like in many other health and care professions its impact is showing positive results. The following chapters in this book will look a little more closely at the knowledge, skills and practice standards that are required to carry out the social work role, suggesting where mindfulness might enhance these areas to the benefit of both the social worker and those who engage with social services.

Take-home message

Mindful social work supports a focus on the present, one that might reduce the need to rely on lessons learned from hindsight.

Takeaways

1. Key points to remember

- Mindfulness is paying attention in a particular way, in the present moment, with openness and without judgement.

- Mindfulness has its roots in religious practice and spirituality but is an ability within all of us and does not need spiritual practice to unveil its potential.

- Scientific research has established a body of work that demonstrates the observable effects mindfulness can have on the brain, including increased self-regulation, cognitive flexibility and focus, reduced anxiety and fear and less rumination, making us happier people as a result.

- Mindfulness is not applicable to everyone in every situation; judgements need to be made about the appropriateness of the mindful approach, particularly when utilising it to address mental health challenges.

- Mindfulness is a natural ally to the social work role and process; its application may lead to increased efficacy in the role.

2. Meditation

A mindful practice beginning: using the guidance below, meditate as long as is comfortable for you.

- Sit in a quiet place with eyes closed; breathe in, becoming aware of the in breath; breathe out, becoming aware of the out breath.

- It is sometimes helpful to concentrate on a point at which the breath touches the body; for example, the sensation of the breath as it enters the nostrils.

- Noticing the breath calms the breath, bringing with it a sense of quiet peacefulness, with mind and body united.

- If thoughts arise, simply let them float past without response and return attention to the breath.

Positive effects can emerge during and after one session of meditation on the breath, but just as the body needs to physically train for a marathon, so the brain needs to be trained to establish good habits of mindfulness and let go of harmful ones. This involves personal commitment, with regular practice staying with the breath even when difficult and challenging thoughts show up. Over time the brain changes its physical structure, enabling the benefits of mindfulness to take hold.

3. A reflection point

Consider the contribution mindfulness could make to your particular social work role: What is the outstanding area where it could help?

 ## 4. Releasing your inner mindful nerd: Topic resource table for self-directed mindful research

Topic	Sources
Understanding mindfulness, its origins and practice	Nhat Hanh, T (1976) *The Miracle of Mindfulness*. Boston: Beacon Press.
	Boyce, B (ed) (2011) *The Mindfulness Revolution*. Boston: Shambhala.
	Henepola Gunaratana, B (2002) *Mindfulness in Plain English*. Sommerville: Wisdom.

Topic	Sources
Mindful benefits for depression	Williams, M, Teasdale, J, Segal, Z and Kabat-Zinn, J (2007) *The Mindful Way Through Depression*. New York: Guilford.
Mindful benefits for anxiety	Orsillo, S and Roemer, L (2011) *The Mindful Way Through Anxiety*. New York: Guildford.
Mindfulness, its positive impact on the brain	Davidson, R J and Begley, S (2012) *The Emotional Life of Your Brain*. New York: Hudson St Press. Siegal, D J (2007) *The Mindful Brain*. New York: Norton.
Mindfulness and creativity	Henriksen, D, Richardson, C and Shack, K (2020) Mindfulness and Creativity: Implications for Thinking and Learning. *Thinking Skills and Creativity*, 37(100689). Penman, D (2021) *Mindfulness for Creativity: Adapt, Create & Thrive in a Frantic World*. London: Piatkus.
Cautionary notes for the use of mindfulness	Britton, W (2019) Can Mindfulness Be Too Much of a Good Thing? The Value of a Middle Way. *Current Opinion in Psychology,* 28: 159–65.
Mindfulness for education	Nhat Hanh, T and Weare, K (2017) *Happy Teachers Change the World: A Guide for Cultivating Mindfulness in Education*. Berkeley: Parallax Press.
Mindfulness for children/young people	Biegal, G (2009) *The Stress Reduction Workbook for Teens*. Oakland: New Harbinger. Kaiser-Greenland, S (2010) *The Mindful Child*. New York: Free Press.

5. Reflection point: The Buddhist eight-fold path for enlightenment

It should be remembered the word 'right' when used in this context does not refer to the right or wrong scenario but relates to balance, to centred regularity rather than a right course of action.

Right view or right understanding: insight into the true nature of reality.

Right intention: unselfish desire to realise enlightenment.

Right speech: using speech compassionately.

Right action: using ethical conduct to manifest compassion.

Right livelihood: making a living through non-harmful means.

Right effort: cultivating wholesome qualities.

Right mindfulness: body and mind awareness.

Right concentration: meditation or other concentrated practice.

(For more on this subject see The Buddhist Centre, nd.)

6. Mindful practice planner

1. It's personal	Your notes
The ability to be mindful exists within all of us; uncovering it and using it to your benefit is a personal experience that can only be led by the self. While there are many guides and tools to help, ultimately it is your own journey, one that is best started by completing a bit of reading or research to help you decide whether you would like to try it, what the outcomes might be for you and how you wish to start being mindful (for example through a mindfulness app or by using a mindful meditation class).	
Your notes	**2. Intention: making yourself a promise**
	If you choose to pursue mindfulness, a good place to start is with an intention. Be clear to yourself what your mindful intention is (for example, to develop mindful skills beneficial to your health and to reduce stress, or to help you to develop increased awareness or a non-judgemental approach to life.

Starting with an intention is always a helpful motivator to continue with practice even if things become challenging. It will therefore be of benefit to write your intention down so that you can revisit it when you need inspiration, but also to reflect on how far you have come when you are further down the mindful path. |

3. Building your own mindful climbing frame

Consider the context in which you will seek to be mindful. Mindful practice can result in changes that others, such as family members, friends and colleagues, may notice. Hopefully, the changes will be positive, but it might be helpful to prepare the way by letting people know that you are embarking on a mindful journey, being open to people joining you if they wished to.

Your notes

Your notes

4. Finding your jumping off point

Decide how you want to practice mindfulness; whether it is through meditation or simple mindful exercises, there are plenty of tools out there to help. But it is important to decide what will fit into your life, how you can manage the development of mindfulness. Don't set yourself up to fail and find yourself in a situation where you are admonishing yourself for not being able to sustain your practice. Above all, be kind to yourself and start with small first steps that you can manage; if you forget your practice or life takes over, don't feel downhearted, just continue where you left off when you put your practice down. Mindfulness takes time; often it can take years to develop a great mindfulness habit, but the important thing is your intent to continue the journey when you encounter bumps in the road.

5. Developing kindness to the self

Prepare yourself for the challenges you might face in your mindful practice: not only the external pressures of adapting your life to accommodate mindfulness, but also the internal experience that can sometimes lead to discomfort. Our daily, busy lives filled with activities can suppress things that we do not want to think about or confront. Mindfulness creates space for difficult subjects to emerge, so one of the keys to practice is to notice thoughts in a non-judgemental way, observing and letting go. Engaging in thoughts with judgement can lead to a spiral of self-critique, one that leads to unhappiness and a letting go of a practice that can lead to peace and happiness.

Your notes

Your notes

6. It's a marathon, not a sprint

The effects of mindfulness practice might be experienced early on, both during quiet moments and in changes of perspective in different aspects of your life. But sustainable peace and contentment come with longevity. Breaking bad habits and establishing mindful ones takes time, and it is important to recognise this. Often at points of struggle it is helpful to seek support from others taking the same journey or to turn to online and textual sources for encouragement and inspiration. Kindness and patience with yourself will help you to stay the course.

References and further reading

Benson, H (1975) *The Relaxation Response*. New York: William Morrow.

Borysenko, J (1987) *Minding the Body, Mending the Mind*. Reading, MA: Addison Wesley.

Brewer, J A, Worhunsky, P D, Gray, J R, Gang, Y, Weber, J and Hedy, K (2011) Meditation Experience is Associated with Differences in Default Mode Network Activity and Connectivity. *PNAS*, 108(50): 20254–9.

Britton, W (2019) Can Mindfulness Be Too Much of a Good Thing? The Value of a Middle Way, *Current Opinion in Psychology*, 28: 159–65.

Cahn, B R and Polich, J (2009) Meditation (Vipassana) and the P3a Event-Related Brain Potential. *International Journal of Psychophysiology*, 72: 51–60.

Carmody, J (2009) Invited Commentary: Evolving Conceptions of Mindfulness in Clinical Settings. *Journal of Cognitive Psychotherapy*, 23(3): 270–80.

Carmody, J and Baer, R A (2008) Relationships between Mindfulness Practice and Levels of Mindfulness, Medical and Psychological Symptoms and Wellbeing in a Mindfulness Stress Reduction Program. *Journal of Behavioural Medicine*, 31(1): 23–33.

Davis, D and Hayes, J A (2011) What Are the Benefits of Mindfulness? *A Practice Review of Psychotherapy Related Research. Psychotherapy*, 48(2): 198–208.

Davison, R J, Kabat-Zinn, J, Schumacher, J, Rozenkranz, M, Muller, D, Santorelli, S F, and Sheridan, J F (2003) Alterations in Brain and Immune Function Produced by Mindfulness Meditation. *Psychosomatic Medicine*, 66: 149–52.

Dusek, J A, Hibberd, P L, Buczynski, B, Benson, H and Zusman, R M (2008) Stress Management versus Lifestyle Modification on Systolic Hypertension and Medication Elimination: A Randomized Trial. *Journal of Alternative and Complementary Medicine*, 14(2): 129–38.

Epel, E, Daubenmier, J, Moskowitz, J T, Folkman, S and Blackburn, E (2009) Can Meditation Slow Rate of Cellular Aging? Cognitive Stress, Mindfulness and Telomeres. Annals of New York Academy of Sciences. *Annals of the New York Academy of Sciences*, 1172(1): 34–53.

Erisman, S M and Roemer, L (2010) A Preliminary Investigation of the Effects of Experimentally Induced Mindfulness on Emotional Responding to File Clips. *Emotion*, 10: 72–82.

Farb, N A S, Anderson, A K, Mayberg, H, Bean, J, McKeon, D and Segal, S V (2010) Minding One's Emotions: Mindfulness Training Alters the Neural Expression of Sadness. *Emotion*, 10: 72–82.

Farb, N A S, Segal, Z C, Mayberg, H, Bean, J, McKeon, D, Fatima, Z and Anderson, A K (2007) Attending to the Present: Mindfulness Meditation Reveals Distinct Neural Modes of Self-Reference. *Social Cognitive and Affective Neuroscience*, 2: 313–22.

Goleman, D and Davison, R J (2010) *Altered Traits: Science Reveals How Meditation Changes your Mind, Brain and Body*. New York: Avery.

Hoffman, S G, Sawyer, A T, Witt, A A and Oh, D (2010) The Effect of Mindfulness-Based Therapy on Anxiety and Depression: A Meta-Analytic Review. *Journal of Consulting and Clinical Psychology,* 78: 169–83.

Holzel, B K, Carmody, J, Vangel, M, Congleton, C, Yerramsetti, T G and Lazar, S (2011) Mindfulness Practice Leads to Increases in Regional Gray Matter Density. *Psychiatry Research: Neuroimaging*, 191(1): 36–43.

Holzel, B K, Carmody, J, Evans, K, Hoje, E, Dusek, J, Morgan, L, Pitman, R and Lazar, S (2010) Stress Reduction Correlates with Structural Changes in the Amygdala. *Social Cognitive and Affective Neuroscience*, 5(1): 11–17.

Judson, A, Brewer, R, Worhunsky P, Gray J, Tang, Y, Weber, J and Kober, H (2011) Meditation Experience is Associated with Differences in Default Mode Network Activity and Connectivity. *PNAS*, 108(50): 20254–9.

Kabat-Zinn, J (1990) *Full Catastrophe Living: Using the Wisdom of your Body and Mind to Face Stress, Pain and Illness*. New York: Delacorte.

Kabat-Zinn, J (1994) *Wherever You Go, There You Are: Mindfulness Meditation in Everyday Life*. New York: Hachette.

Lazar, W W, Kerr, C E, Wasserman, R H, Gray, J R, Greve, D N, Treadway, M T and Fischl, B (2005) Meditation Experience is Associated with Increased Cortical Thickness. *Neuro Report for Rapid Communication of Neuroscience Research*, 16: 1893–7.

Logan, S L (2014) Meditation, Mindfulness and Social Work. *Social Work Journal for Women*. [online] Available at: https://oxfordre.com/socialwork/abstract/10.1093/acrefore/9780199975839.001.0001/acrefore-9780199975839-e-981 (accessed 9 September 2022).

Nhat Hanh, T (nd) Plum Village. [online] https://plumvillage.org (accessed 18 August 2022).

Ortner, C N M, Kilner, S J and Zelazo, P D (2007) Mindfulness Meditation and Reduced Emotional Interference on a Aognitive Task. *Motivation and Emotion*, 31: 271–83.

Purser, R (2019) *McMindfulness: How Mindfulness Became the New Capitalist Spirituality*. New York: Repeater Books.

Purser, R E, Forbes, D and Burke, A (eds) (2019) *Handbook of Mindfulness: Culture, Context, and Social Engagement*. Switzerland: Springer Link.

Ridgeon, L (2003) *Major Religions of the World*. New York: Taylor & Francis.

Roemer, L, Orsillo, S M and Salters-Pedneault, K (2008) Efficacy of an Acceptance-Based Behaviour Therapy for Generalised Anxiety Disorder: Evaluation in a Randomised Controlled Trial. *Journal of Consulting and Clinical Psychology*, 76(6): 1083–9.

Science Daily (2009) Meditation May Increase Grey Matter. 13 May. [online] Available at: www.sciencedaily.com/releases/2009/05/090512134655.htm (accessed 8 September 2022).

Teasdale, J D and Chaskalson, M (2011) How Does Mindfulness Transform Suffering? I: The Nature and Origins of Dukkha. *Contemporary Buddhism*, 12(1): 89–102.

The Buddhist Centre (nd) Noble Eightfold Path. [online] Available at: https://thebuddhistcentre.com/text/noble-eightfold-path (accessed 9 September 2022).

Trousselard, M, Stiler, D, Claverie, D and Canini, F (2014) The History of Mindfulness Put to the Test of Current Scientific Data: Unresolved Questions. *Encephale*, 40(6): 474–80.

Williams, M (2018) *Mindfulness*. London: NHS. [online] Available at: www.nhs.uk/mental-health/self-help/tips-and-support/mindfulness (accessed 18 August 2022).

Wolkin, J (2015) How the Brain Changes When You Meditate. [online] Available at: www.mindful.org/how-the-brain-changes-when-you-meditate (accessed 6 September 2022).

Chapter 2

The mindful social worker: living your best social work life

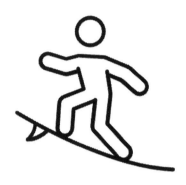

You can't stop the waves, but you can learn how to surf
(Kabat-Zinn, 1990)

There are many different reasons why people choose to become social workers, but they invariably will involve self-evaluation of personal experiences, skills and values that develop a commitment to help support others. Usually social work recruits are also motivated by desires to reduce inequality, to protect the most vulnerable and to enable people to enjoy a good quality of life. However, like other caring professions, the role is subject to high levels of pressure that if unchecked can accumulate to cause both mental and physical harm to self; getting the health balance right for social workers is an ever-increasing challenge.

Historically overlooked, but perhaps now becoming of greater importance, is the realisation that the social work professional needs to take care of self not only for their own sake but also to be effective in the support of others. Effective practice for the long term needs to recognise the imperative for social workers' to 'put their own oxygen mask on first' to sustain their own well-being in a manner that enables them to fully support those they work with.

Mindfulness has become a popular reference tool for both personal and professional self-care within the caring professions – health and social work in particular – due in most part to its effectiveness in supporting well-being, while also having the potential to reduce the impact of overexposure to trauma, compassion fatigue and burnout (Crowder and Sears, 2017, p 17). Positive correlations have been found between those exercising a social work role who practice mindfulness and an increased social work ability to cope with stressful situations (McGarrigle and Walsh, 2011; Gockel and Deng, 2016). It is also encouraging to note that the benefits of mindfulness in this professional arena appear to extend beyond the immediate; social workers and social work students who practise mindfulness report additional longer-term experiences of peace, contentment and happiness.

One social worker involved in a mindful study reported that mindfulness *'encouraged a dramatic positive mind shift and caused me to prioritise life priorities and gave me confidence to be my authentic self with happier life outcomes'* (Roulston et al, 2018, pp 164–5). This chapter seeks to capture the advantages a mindful practice can have for those working in the social work field, with opportunities for reflection about the application of mindfulness as a pillar of support in an ever-changing, challenging professional field. Focusing on the quality mindfulness holds to help restore that much sought-after work–life balance that can elude those who work within such a physically and emotionally demanding job.

This chapter will include:

The elephant in the room: stress

Leaning into stress

Signs of stress

Putting your own oxygen mask on first

Ordinary magic

Changing the narrative

The elephant in the room: stress

 A recent YouGov survey of social workers, undertaken in 2019, discovered many participants experienced a great deal to be positive about the social work role. Among the highlights there were reports of social workers who enjoyed and valued their job, felt able to make a difference and were inspired by their organisations to be the best they could be, reports that illustrate there is a best social work life to be lived. However, the same survey found the inevitable presence of a high degree of stress among the workforce. Over 85 per cent of participants reported stress; a significant number also identified as having low morale, particularly in relation to the negative media perception of the role. These findings concur with a similarly recent summary of work-related health and safety statistics for Great Britain (HSE, 2019), which placed social work in the highest group for work-related stress, depression and anxiety, across all professions reviewed.

Stress is ever present in the social work role but is frequently not explicitly acknowledged, and is mentioned in social work professional conversations but without a clear strategy to address the stress characteristics that go with social work practice. A survey conducted by Plymouth University (Beer and Asthana, 2016) revealed concerning results not only in relation to stress levels among the social work profession but also in relation to the coping behaviours used to offset stress. Participants in this study highlighted the use of emotional eating, alcohol and in some cases drugs as a means of coping. Many reported difficulties with sleeping, feelings of emotional exhaustion and concern about impending burnout. A significant proportion felt overwhelmed at work. All of these factors present a worrying picture not only of the health of the workforce but also of the quality of work that people enduring such pressure are able to deliver to service users.

> *There is little debate over social work's status as a stressful profession. Social Worker's practice in an increasingly difficult environment characterised by rising demands, diminishing resources and negative scrutiny from the media.*
>
> (Beer and Asthana, 2016)

Stress is no surprise in social work, but it is surprising that within the workplace setting scant attention is paid to how these stress factors are addressed.

The dynamics of social work

Social work has a particular dynamic: it is demanding, rewarding and challenging; it can provide a deep sense of fulfilment when supporting change that results in better outcomes for service users, while also exposing the social worker to increased levels of anxiety and pressure when things are not going well. It is a complex role that requires the social worker to negotiate intervention both at an individual level and at a societal level in the form of social justice.

> *two interconnected fronts, a focus of change at the community and societal level, and a focus of change on the individual level.*
>
> (McLaughlin, 2002, p 189)

This balancing act is further complicated by the growth of managerial requirements over recent years, particularly the adoption of managerial performance approaches that require documented evidence of practice. This dichotomy of demand between value-based relational social work and evidence-based performance can bring both internal and external conflict to the practitioner who needs to reconcile both to daily working life. A picture emerges of the social work experience as one of strong emotional intensity that tests physical and psychological well-being to the full extent of personal limits (Logan, 2014).

The distinct dynamics of the social work role serve to make the profession a complex one to navigate; indeed, in trying to do so, many of the internalised conflicts begin to emerge in practice, noticeably through compassion fatigue or burnout, both of which are regularly spoken of as an inevitable part of the role. Burnout has been described as a type of *'emotional exhaustion'*, with a loss of *'a sense of mission in one's work'* (Conrad and Kellar-Guenther, 2006). It is identified as a condition that results in a disengagement or distancing from the work, with an obvious detrimental implication for those that need help. Equally, the emergence of compassion fatigue, resulting from overexposure to trauma, can mean a loss of the ability to stay with the difficulties of others at a time when one's presence is most needed. In effect, pressures on social workers can lead to dehumanisation in a humane profession (Davies and Collings, 2008).

Not just getting by

When asked, most social workers confirm that they enter the profession with aspirations of being able to 'make a difference' (YouGov, 2019) and realise ideals of equality, social change and care. The capacity to achieve this aim is present within the profession, confirmed by practitioners who identify opportunities to make a positive impact and improve people's lives. The presence of stress can sometimes obscure or hinder the actualisation of such opportunities.

Stress exists within all professions, indeed in work in general, its presence is part of daily living and necessary to galvanise activity, creativity and adaptability. However, when it reaches debilitating levels, social workers can be reduced to only just 'getting by' at work rather than living a best social work life. While stress cannot be eliminated, nor should it be, it can be managed or responded to in a way that transforms it into an increasingly benign presence, offsetting its more negative long-term effects.

Mindfulness has emerged as one of a combination of practices that can help to bring stress into manageable proportions. If utilised in a supportive, organisational workplace context, it has demonstrably improved the quality of employees' working lives. A practice accessed repeatedly within the caring professions as a means of moving beyond reaction to stress to control of its impact. In many occupations across the world, mindfulness has become a golden thread that links both organisation and individual in the process of calming the mind and developing a kinder way of living that gives greater space for positivity, peace and well-being. '*Without mindfulness, we can't help ourselves, or our loved ones, or succeed in our workplace*' (Nhat Hanh, 2007). Within a caring profession, the progress of social work toward a best professional life, must begin with self-care, because if they are unable to care for their own self, how can the practitioner advise others to do the same?

Leaning into stress

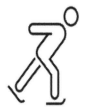 It seems counterintuitive, but in order to respond well to stress, particularly through the use of mindfulness, its character must be understood, to enable the mindful social worker to recognise when stress is occurring and, in the spirit of all social work action, prevent its escalation. The mindful social worker will need to lean into stress, increasing awareness of when it is taking place and noticing if it is a prolonged experience in order to meet it with an intelligent, mindful response rather than a mindless spiral of tension.

Keeping in mind the scientific research that highlights that short-term periods of stress are acceptable and often useful in driving action or adaptability, while also retaining awareness of the detrimental long-term influence of stress on health outcomes, will help to increase one's awareness of the personal stress reaction. This referencing of information can also act as reminder to help one prioritise stress management in self-care, particularly when measured against the poor health outcomes from exposure to high levels of long-term pressure: cardiovascular disease, diabetes, cancer, auto-immune syndromes, mental disorders, depression and anxiety (Koolhass et al, 2011; Mariottie et al, 2015; Mental Health Foundation, 2021).

It should be noted that everyone responds to stress differently and experiences different levels of stress even when faced with the same challenges. It is the perception of a threat that acts as the initiator of the brain's stress response. One person might find a situation stressful, whereas another may not experience symptoms at all, and this can be attributed to a variety of factors, which might include: self-confidence, familiarity with the presenting pressure, life experience, skill and know-ledge relating to the presenting issue. The rate at which the brain returns to balance can also depend on these factors, while the balance may also be interrupted by maladaptive responses to stress, such as alcohol intake, overeating or excessive exercise.

Mindful practice enables the mindful social worker to increase their awareness of self at work, to notice any individual changes in behaviour, mood or activity that could give rise to concern, perhaps experiencing certain situations as particularly stressful, and to noticing the source of stress that needs greater attention. Consider the following signs of stress described below as part of understanding stress as it manifests in self (adapted from the Mental Health Foundation, nd; NHS, nd, Mindfulness. org, 2012).

Signs of stress

This is not an exhaustive list, and it should be borne in mind that many of the signs of stress can also be indicative of other medical conditions that might require consultation with a professional. However, the signs of stress below are an important weather balloon in judging where individual stress levels are.

anxiety	headaches	withdrawing
irritability	nausea	snapping
fear	indigestion	indecision
aggression	bowel discomfort	tearfulness
sadness	hyperventilating	increased sleeping
frustration	palpitations	insomnia
helplessness	shallow breathing	excessive behaviour, eg, alcohol use
depression	sweating	aches and pains

Mindful point of reflection

Pause and take a moment to consider the signs of stress, and complete a mind-and-body check to find out if stress exists within your life. Reflect on whether it is at an acceptable level or whether those aches and pains caused by tension have been there too long. Undertaking this exercise can help to maintain a mindful practice of self-monitoring, providing the ability to make small adjustments to prevent a rise in stress levels.

There are of course life situations that will predictably increase stress levels, and it is good to be aware of these in order to put in place coping strategies, including a mindful approach. The following are recognised points of possible excessive pressure where mindful reflection can help in preparing or creating change in order to manage the impact of these significant events.

changes in job	financial difficulties	conflict at home or work
changes in work conditions	high loan or mortgage payments	divorce/separation
changes in work hours	changes in sleeping patterns	challenges with children
changes in routine	changes in eating habits	increase in arguments
changes in responsibilities at work	challenging health conditions	movement of home or accommodation

(Adapted from Holmes and Rache, 1967; Cohen et al, 1983)

While these are challenging events that can often be foreseen, they are ones that most people experience at some point during life. But there are also unanticipated stressful events that defy preparation. These are perhaps most relevant to social work, a role that encounters unpredictability every day in practice, much of which involves tearing up plans and starting again. Adding any of the above-described personal life changes into the mix can create a toxic situation that will test even the most relaxed professional to their tolerance limits.

Historically, the longstanding stress test scale of Holmes and Rache (1967), alongside that of Cohen et al (1983), has provided a fairly comprehensive view of where stressors might lie. However, neither test has anticipated the ubiquitous nature of technology in the modern world, which can be both a help and very much a hindrance and a rich source of stress for the human condition. The technology-fuelled immediacy of competing demands that take place within one's work and personal lives can add yet more complexity to the day, alongside the enticement of social media which can distract a person for hours while other tasks and work build up to an overwhelming scale.

Additionally, surprise events, such as the Covid-19 pandemic, only serve to accentuate tensions in life further; in essence, well-being is fragile when pitted against the mental load of dealing with the unpredictable. The case for self-care has surely been made over recent decades, and nowhere is it more needed than in the social work profession. Organisational and individual action to manage stress can help social work practitioners to move beyond just getting by in social work practice towards achieving a best social work life that encompasses the original intentions of those who choose the profession: making a difference, and feeling valued and encouraged by employers to be a best professional self.

Take-home message

The only thing that can be reliably expected is the unexpected, mindfulness helps the practitioner accept, understand and respond to this state.

Putting your own oxygen mask on first

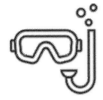 People who work in the caring professions too often prioritise the needs of others before their own, and social work is no exception; but the question remains as to whether such self-sacrifice hinders individual effect-iveness both in personal and work life. Social work has accepted a culture of burnout for many years, a situation that can lead to high turnover of staff as well as increased absence due to sickness, culminating in a reduction of professionals' ability to carry out very complex, demanding work. By the law of diminishing returns, if social workers do not prioritise self-care, their ability to provide support for others will become compromised, and they will experience a personal cost to their well-being.

Prioritising your own wellbeing is not selfish but vital if you are going to be able to sustain best practice in these difficult times.

(Grant and Kinman, 2020)

In recent years there has been an increasing focus on work–life balance, with many organisations emphasising the importance of self-care and often creating work environments to support employees to adopt wellness strategies. Mindfulness, within a supportive work context, is just such a research-proven strategy that can enable the professional social worker to meet the inevitability of stress on terms that empower them to respond well, an approach that helps to preserve peace of mind while also creating space to let in the things that help create a best social work life: the recognition of success; a sense of humour; a balanced perspec-tive; an understanding that all things change; knowing when support is needed and when colleagues, friends and service users need extra help. Self-care through mindfulness forms a complementary foundation to the employer's duty of care, but social workers should be alert to the fact that mindful self-care might also in itself include advocating for an increasingly mindful culture in the workplace to the benefit of all.

Mindful point of reflection

Take the opportunity to consider how your workplace might change through the introduction of mindfulness, and how you and your colleagues could advocate for such change.

Ordinary magic

 Masten (2009) uses the term 'ordinary magic' to describe the power of small routine steps to produce great results in well-being. It is also relevant to the benefits that mindfulness can bring. A mindful meditation routine, however short, undertaken regularly can yield significant changes for the better. The challenge is to both begin and sustain the mindful journey. There is always a point at which the reading or researching needs to stop and the mindful practice needs to begin, as mindfulness is a personal experiential process that is unique to each individual; description can never accurately portray the experience.

The research bit

Social work, involving interactions with all that it is to be human, is a profession that demands resilience in order to maintain both effectiveness and longevity. Mindful practice in social work can form the foundation of resilience in order to meet the demands of the role; research in this area seems to agree.

Studies undertaken with both social workers in training and more experienced practitioners indicate mindfulness can make a positive contribution to professionals' ability to cope (Ying, 2008; McGarrigle and Walsh, 2011; Gockel and Deng, 2016). Participants within these studies were able to give present attention to their experience of stress, enabling evasive action to be taken to mitigate its effects, reducing stress levels to more acceptable states. Developing this ability gives practitioners the potential to develop greater objectivity regarding work pressures, and allows them to seek help earlier and in a much more targeted way through identified supervision or management channels.

In particular a study involving social work students highlighted the relationship between mindfulness practice and a reduction in student anxiety and stress alongside enhanced awareness of emotional reactivity, the latter enabling self-action to be taken to better regulate emotions (Howie et al, 2016; Roulston et al, 2018; McCusker, 2019). The increased awareness of self as a result of mindful practice also produced acknowledgement of the need for self-care, instigating exploration of ongoing coping strategies that could maintain a much greater level of homeostasis of the body and mind. The strategies deployed included a continuation of mindfulness, which improved sleep activity, and making reference to the breath at times of stress, restoring calm to imbalance. Kinman et al (2020) advocate referencing the mindful state of awareness at regular points during the day by checking in with a watch and reconnecting with the breath as a way of maintaining a constancy of calm when challenged by daily activity. Indeed, this approach mirrors the Buddhist practice of using a bell to signal the need to bring awareness to the present.

Research has recognised the important perceptual shift that mindfulness can achieve. It is understood that it is the perception of stress that triggers the fight-or-flight response in the brain. This explains why individuals all have different stress responses to the same situation: one person's stress response is not another person's. However, a study conducted into mindfulness practice among social work students found participants reported a feeling of improvement in their quality of life as a result of mindfulness, despite a continuation of their usual stress levels (Bonifas and Napoli, 2014).

In support of social work kindness to self, mindfulness practice has the capacity to increase compassion in social work while also building strengths to combat the familiar sense of burnout experienced by so many social work professionals (Crowder and Sears, 2017; McCusker, 2019). Notably, a direct correlation between high levels of compassion fatigue and lower levels of mindfulness practice has been found among social work students, demonstrating a positive link between mindfulness and sustained empathetic social work intervention (Brown et al, 2015). This would suggest mindfulness is key in developing compassion for both self and others.

However, perhaps mindfulness's greatest significance for social work practice is the safe, quiet space it provides for the reconciliation of both professional and private lives in a place of calm balance, reducing the bombardment of pressure and information to silence (McGarrigle and Walsh, 2011). This is in fact best illustrated by a social work participant in a mindful study who described meditation as '*my secret space*' (Kinman et al, 2019).

Practice examples

The following are examples of organisations that have recognised the value of mindfulness and its implementation in the work setting:

- *the Australian Association of Social Workers's Social Work Yoga and Mindfulness Practice Group;*

- *university of Buffalo, New York, School of Social Work's self-care starter kits that include mindfulness resources;*

- *the European Union's training of climate change staff in meditation, seeking to take mindfulness off cushion into hard politics (Booth, 2022);*

- *the United Nations' goal to create a global mindful community through their Mindful Living Network.*

Changing the narrative

 Mindfulness is being integrated into the workplace at both a global and national scale, establishing its pedigree as a very real method of support for those facing difficult situations. The practice does not remove problems but creates perspective shifts that enable different interpretations of situations, leading to better coping strategies and (dare it be said) greater enjoyment of work. Mindfulness opens possibilities for changing the narrative of work, leading to an increasingly positive experience that impacts the outcomes of the work activity, progress that begins with the establishment of regular mindful interludes. Resources are available throughout this book and in the Resource hut at the end to help engender such mindful moments or longer periods of meditation in a way that suits each person's approach and lifestyle. But the important point to remember is: less talk and more experience through practice in order for mindfulness to become an integral part of life rather than just another thing to do.

> *Self-care is not something to do just in your spare time or on vacation. It is a disposition, attitude, or ongoing state of body and mind.*
>
> (Cox and Steiner, 2013)

A useful way to start living a best social work life is to take some mindful moments to consider self within the social work professional context. Working day to day in a busy environment does not always enable reflection on one's individual social work career or on the best way to live the experience. Conducting a mindful review based on the tools available in the 'Takeaways' section at the end of this chapter can help to clarify one's aspirations for the future and the intention to achieve positive change for people that come into contact with social work services, while also helping to change a narrative from one of pressure and burnout to one of creativity, kindness and wisdom both for one's own well-being and the well-being of those around you.

Many social work participants in mindful studies report a sense of reconnecting with their inner self, particularly with compassion and kindness, reducing the drive to be all things to all people and recognising and accepting limitations. In turn, this provides benefits beyond meditation into everyday life (off cushion benefits), adding wisdom to one's engagement with others. These insights can be the first steps to acknowledging the need for change in which there is advocacy for good working conditions and mindful understanding of when and how support is needed in order to maintain good professional health, and consequently good personal health.

As mindful practice deepens, it can enable more profound contemplation on the enactment of the social work role itself, raising the prospect of living a best social work life. The creation of mindful distance from daily reactivity to the demands of practice exercised through managerial and organisational expectations facilitates the individual evaluation of career-role aspirations. This enables a comparison to be made between the experience of fulfilling the social work role alongside personal/professional values, with the expectations of working within a social work career. This identifies the prospect of reaching greater harmony between the individuals' expectations of a best social work life and those of employer organisations. Mindfulness offers the chance to take regular, objective work-health checks, resulting in adjustments to ensure that the movement towards a best social work professional life is possible.

Above all, mindfulness offers an opportunity for social workers to reconnect with their vocation, the meaning and authenticity of the role, to dial down the predominance of stress and dial up the awareness of all that is good about the role, creating a gateway to '*bring themselves home*' (Doxtdator, 2012)

> *Mindfulness may offer social workers a means to return to a place of authenticity and meaning, returning the sense of vocation that initially called many to social work, allowing social workers, a pathway to 'bring themselves home'.*
>
> (Doxtdator, 2012)

Ultimately, both qualitative and quantitative information suggest mindfulness might be a very worthwhile means of reaching a best social work life.

Takeaways

1. Key Points to remember

- Mindfulness can help social workers meet the pressures of the job on their own terms, facilitating greater control over its effects on mind and body.

- By recognising personal signs of stress through mindful self-monitoring, steps can be taken to initiate a relaxation response.

- Self-care for social workers prioritises meeting their own needs as well as the needs of others.

- Mindfulness is ordinary magic; small steps in regular practice produce greater well-being results.

- Mindfulness allows social workers to interrupt stressful experience, replacing it with a best social work life that returns to the original intent and values of the role.

2. Check out your mindful approach

This list is not a diagnostic tool but an opportunity for reflection on how many of these behaviours feature in your working day, and if you are unhappy with their frequency, it may support your intention to embark on a mindful practice to bring them back under your control.

- I think about work or personal issues all the time during my commute, without noticing my journey.

- I am anxious about getting through my workload during the day.

- I leave meetings or contacts without noticing my travel or remembering what people have told me.

- I sit in meetings or during visits preoccupied with the emails on my device at the same time as I am taking part in the contact.

- I forget to meet my physical needs during work, such as hydration or eating.

- I do not have regular breaks away from my desk during the day.

- I am easily distracted from my work by emails and notifications.

- My mind wanders to the internet or office conversation frequently.

- I easily forget people's names or what they have told me during the day.

- There are few moments in my day when I pause to reflect on what I am doing.

- I do not make space for creative thought during the day.

- I do not recognise and acknowledge my emotions or feelings as they occur during the day.

- I have difficulty relaxing at the end of the day, and struggle to manage the thoughts running through my brain.

- I continue to think about work when it is time to sleep, and this disrupts my sleep.

The more of these statements you tick off, the more it suggests a mindful approach might be beneficial if you wish to change these behaviours.

3. Body scan for relaxation

The use of body-checking or scanning techniques can be a good way to establish a mindful position in the present. It is a particularly helpful practice for establishing the mind-body connection. Time spent body scanning, paying attention to problematic areas, provides daily living benefits, helping one to notice when tension is emerging in the body and to engage a relaxation response to soften the affected areas.

How to start

Body scanning involves directing attention to parts of the body. Nothing else is needed. As you bring attention to specific areas, notice the area soften under awareness.

- Find a quiet place to sit or lie down with your eyes closed.

- Start with the top of the head, move down through the face to the neck, bringing particular attention to the forehead and any tension in the jaw as you move down.

- Extend to the shoulders, bringing awareness to any tension to either side.

- Travel along each arm to the wrist, hand and fingers.

- Gently return to the chest, moving down to the waist. Travel down each leg to the feet and toes.

- Bring attention to the back of the body, starting with the back of legs, moving up through to waist, back, shoulders.

- Return to the neck and back of head.

Body scanning results in a calmer, relaxed body that in turn brings peace to the mind. Allow some deep breaths before returning sensation to the body. Start by wiggling your toes and fingers, gently moving to slowly open the eyes.

Take a few moments to notice how your body feels when it is relaxed. This will help you recognise when tension requires a response. The body-scan technique, if practised regularly, can be used in short sessions during the day to notice and combat any pain or tension in our lives. It can also be a useful way to relax at night to induce better sleep.

Guided body-check meditations can be found at HeadSpace.com and Mindful.org. There are also a number of recordings that can be live-streamed from YouTube and iTunes.

4. A mindful approach to living a best social work life

Change your narrative.

Take some moments to complete this mindful application tool. It can be used regularly to reset your short-term social work life or for the long-term direction of your aspirations.

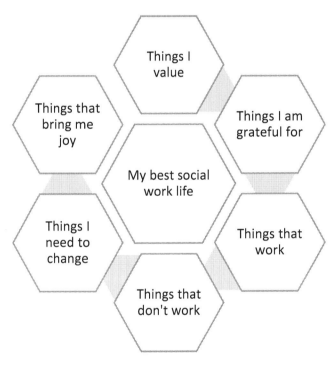

Figure 1.1 Change your narrative

What are the next steps that need to be taken?

5. Six mindful support pillars for reflection

Use the blank space in this table to record your reminders or what you will do to make sure you honour these mindful principles to live a good life.

Patience Living life in each moment; letting change occur in its own time; noticing differences as they occur; meditation is whatever arises.	
	Non-judgement Resisting the human tendency to leap to judgement; allowing experience of things as they really are, without anticipation by the mind.
Trust Confidence in self, with faith in the ability of mindfulness to enhance well-being for self and those around you.	
	Non-striving There is no success or failure, there is just mindful practice; experience is unique to the individual, no competition exists; do not grasp at success but allow it to unfold at its own pace.
Acceptance Accept whatever occurs, accessing life as it is, not how we would like it to be.	
	Letting go Do not grasp or hold on to things, experiences or feelings; let them go, understanding that change is constant.

(adapted from Kabat-Zinn, 1990)

References and further reading

Beer, O and Asthana, S (2016) *How Stress Impacts Social Workers and How They're Trying to Cope*. Plymouth: University of Plymouth.

Bonifas, R P and Napoli, M (2014) Mindfully Increasing Quality of Life: A Promising Curriculum for MSW Students. *Social Work Education*, 27(8): 837–52.

Booth, R (2022) EU Officials Being Trained to Meditate to Help Fight Climate Crisis. *The Guardian*. [online] Available at: www.theguardian.com/world/2022/may/04/eu-bureaucrats-being-trained-meditate-help-fight-climate-crisis#:~:text=Brussels%20officials%20are%20being%20trained,cushion%E2%80%9D%20and%20into%20hard%20politics (accessed 18 August 2022).

Brown, K W, Creswell, J D and Ryan, M (2015) Introduction the Evolution of Mindfulness Science. In Brown, K W, Creswell, J D and Ryan, M (eds) *Handbook of Mindfulness* (pp 1–6). New York: Guilford Publications.

Cohen, S, Kamarch, T and Mermelstein, R (1983) A Global Measure of Perceived Stress. *Journal of Health and Social Behaviour*, 24: 385–96.

Conrad, D and Kellar-Guenther, Y (2006) Compassion Fatigue, Burnout and Compassion Satisfaction among Colorado Child Protection Workers. *Child Abuse & Neglect*, 30(10): 1071–80.

Cox, K and Steiner, S (2013) *Self care in Social Work: A Guide for Practitioners*. North Carolina: NASW Press.

Crowder, R and Sears, A (2017) Building Resilience in Social Workers: An Exploratory Study on the Impacts of a Mindfulness-Intervention. *Australian Social Work*, 70(1): 17–29.

Davies, L and Collings, S (2008) Emotional Knowledge for Child Welfare Practice. Rediscovering Our Roots. *Smith College Studies in Social Work*, 78(1): 7–26.

Doxtdator, M L (2012) *Mindfulness: Helping Social Workers 'Bring Themselves Home'*. Ontario: McMaster School of Social Work, McMaster University.

Garrett, P M (2016) Questioning Tales of 'Ordinary Magic': Resilience and Neo-Liberal Reasoning. *British Journal of Social Work*, 46(7): 1909–25.

Gockel, A and Deng, X (2016) Mindfulness Training as Social Work Pedagogy: Exploring Benefits, Challenges, and Issues for Consideration in Integrating Mindfulness into Social Work Education. *Journal of Religion & Spirituality in Social Work: Social Thought*, 35(3): 222–44.

Grant, L and Kinman, G (2020) *Developing Emotional Resilience and Well-Being: A Practical Guide for Social Workers*. [online] Available at: https://mark allenassets.blob.core.windows.net/communitycare/2020/04/Community-Care-Inform-emotional-resilience-guide.pdf (accessed 18 August 2022).

Holmes, T H and Rache, R H (1967) The Social Readjustment Rating Scale. *Journal of Psychosomatic Research*, 11: 213–18.

Howie, J, Innes, D and Harvey, P (2016) Promoting Conscious Competence by Introducing Mindfulness to Social Worker Students. *Journal or Practice Teaching and Learning*, 14(1): 88–104.

HSE (Health and Safety Executive) (2019) Summary Statistics for Great Britain 2019. [online] Available at: www.hse.gov.uk/statistics/overall/hssh1819.pdf (accessed 9 September 2022).

Kabat-Zinn, J (1990) *Full Catastrophe Living: Using the Wisdom of your Body and Mind to Face Stress, Pain and Illness*. New York: Random House.

Kabat-Zinn, J (1994) *Wherever You Go, There You Are: Mindfulness Meditation in Everyday Life*. New York: Hachette.

Kinman, G, Grant, L and Kelly, S (2020) 'It's My Secret Space' The Benefits of Mindfulness for Social Workers. *The British Journal of Social Work*, 50(3): 758–77.

Koolhass, J M et al (2011) Stress Revisited: A Critical Evaluation of the Stress Concept. *Neuroscience & Biobehavioral Reviews*, 35(5): 1291–301.

Logan, S L (2014) Meditation, Mindfulness and Social Work. Social Work Journal for Women. [online] Available at: https://oxfordre.com/socialwork/abstract/10.1093/acrefore/9780199975839.001.0001/acrefore-9780199975839-e-981 (accessed 9 September 2022).

Mariottie, A (2015) The Effects of Chronic Stress on Health: New Insights into Molecular Mechanisms of the Brain Body Communication. *Future Science*, 1(3). doi:10.4155/fso.15.21.

Masten, A (2009) Ordinary Magic: Lessons Learned from Research on Resilience in Human Development. *Education Canada*, 49(3): 28–32.

McCusker, P (2019) Critical Mindfulness in Social Work: Self-Care as Anti-Oppressive Practice, Theory and Pedagogy in the Journey from Social Work Student to Social Worker. PhD Thesis. Glasgow Caledonian University.

McGarrigle, T and Walsh, C A (2011) Mindfulness, Self-Care, and Wellness in Social Work. *Social Thought*, 30(3): 212–33.

McLaughlin, A M (2002) Social Work's Legacy: Irreconcilable Differences? *Clinical Social Work Journal*, 30(2): 187–98.

McLaughlin, A M (2011) Exploring Social Justice for Clinical Social Work Practice. *Smith College Studies in Social Work*, 81(2–3): 234–51.

Mental Health Foundation (nd) Stress. [online] Available at: www.mentalhealth.org.uk/explore-mental-health/a-z-topics/stress (accessed 28 September 2022).

Mindfulness.org (2012) Stress and Mindfulness. [online] Available at: www.mindful.org/stress-and-mindfulness (accessed 28 September 2022).

Nhat Hanh, T (2007) *The Art of Power.* London: HarperCollins.

NHS (nd) Feeling Stressed? [online] Available at: www.nhs.uk/every-mind-matters/mental-health-issues/stress (accessed 28 September 2022).

Roulston, A, Mongomery, L, Campbell, A and Davidson, G (2018) Exploring the Impact of Mindfulness on Mental Wellbeing, Stress, and Resilience of Undergraduate Social Work Students. *Social Work Education*, 37(2): 157–72.

Ying, Y W (2008) Variation in Personal Competence and Mental Health Between Entering and Graduating NSW Students: The Contribution of Mindfulness. *Journal of Religion and Spirituality in Social Work, Social Thought*, 27(4): 405–22.

YouGov (2019) *A Report on Social Work in England, Executive Summary*. London: YouGov.

Chapter 3

Mindful communication

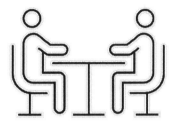

When you talk, you are only repeating what you already know. But if you listen, you may learn something new.

(Dalai Lama)

This chapter will look at how mindfulness can make an important contribution to the scaffolding of support for good communication in social work. Consideration of the act of being present in the moment identifies the benefits of mindfulness in its serving to enhance work in partnership with people to promote their well-being.

Mindful communication involves being present in the conversation, undisturbed, with focused attention on what is being communicated, checking not only verbal messages but also non-verbal cues and the mood in the room. It enhances one's empathetic response to people, valuing them as individuals, honouring their conversations with respect and dignity. Mindful communication is the bridge through which accurate assessments and interventions can be made in a way that builds on a given person's strengths and forms partnerships across families and communities to reach positive outcomes in a person-centred way.

This chapter will include:

The simple yet complex act of communication

Let's talk

What are you trying to say?

Paralanguage

The full picture

Listening

Listening well

The difference between hearing and listening

The simple yet complex act of communication

 Social workers are expected to be the chameleons of communication, adapting language and behaviour to a wide
variety of situations, including the professional arenas of
meetings, court and conferences, while also encompassing
direct communication with service users, groups and communities; the
latter of a style that avoids jargon and gets the message across. But the
role is not only about delivering messages; it is also about listening and
responding in these same ever-changing contexts. Add to this individuals'
expectations, distress, anger and sometimes great happiness that a
longed-for service will be delivered, and we can begin to see the mammoth
task that lies ahead for social workers whose role is to negotiate
partnerships that deliver positive change for people accessing services.

Communication is the bedrock of effective practice and the main tool
through which intervention can succeed or fail. It is unsurprising that
social work is thought to have been the first profession to recognise the
importance of communication as a skill and its link to good social work
practice (Nelsen, 1980). If social workers are unable to facilitate good communication with the people they are supporting, any help is destined to
be badly received and misdirected and will ultimately lead to failure.

Social work is a relationship-based profession that is dependent on
collaboration with agreed goals across partnerships between all those
engaged, including adults, children, communities and professionals. Such
partnerships are formed from a baseline of trust and respect, commod-
ities that are built from good, effective communication, and are easily

broken by the wrong word or by messages delivered in the wrong way, particularly when working with vulnerable people, who may already distrust the service, or people who have had bad experiences in the past and are anxious about social work intervention.

Social work communication is inevitably hampered by the perceived and very real disparity between the authority and power of service users and social workers, who hold decision-making capabilities that can have significant life-changing effects on a person's life (for example, the removal of a child from parents or the decision to restrict an adult's freedom). This imbalance serves to remind the profession that communication needs to be clear and unbiased, with reflection on the nature of what is being said and heard. Building strong relationships both with service users and professionals can be an arduous task that takes care and commitment, and it can easily be damaged with lack of care in communication. Communication, therefore, should not be a stream of verbal information that tumbles from the busy mind, but a mindful act of clarity. Thompson (2020) highlights several barriers to keep in mind when communicating; they include: authority, age, gender, ability, personality and class. These factors can become a point of reflection for social workers to consider their impact on one's own professional communication and the communication of others. Keeping them in mind, as Thompson suggests, enables mindful awareness of the role they play in effective messaging in individual, meeting-based and virtual contexts, while also creating a framework for the consideration of factors that need to be overcome in order to achieve full understanding.

Humans are born with the innate trait of communicativeness as a means of meeting needs, either individually or through group/community co-operation. Our first communications are non-verbal signalling through sounds or physical signs such as smiles or frowns. As we grow, communication develops into the spoken word, while non-verbal indicators are retained to enhance understanding. The need to be understood, therefore, compels us to communicate; indeed if someone is non-communicative, we take that as a cause of concern for their well-being. But the various layers of communication make understanding others and being understood a difficult act. Particularly when virtual aspects of communication, such as social media, email and so forth, add an additional layer to this complexity. Communication includes both giving and receiving; mindful competency in both these aspects can serve to enhance full comprehension within this vital activity.

Let's talk

Consideration of verbal communication alone serves to highlight the things that can lead to misunderstanding, indicating the importance of present-moment awareness to communication and understanding. As humans, there is a constant stream of chatter or thought in our minds that often translates into a continual stream of external verbal communication with little thought regarding its impact on others. As social workers, the words we use, the sentences constructed to deliver thoughts, advice and information, are central to engagement with the other person. Strengths-based, solution-focused approaches to social work serve to illustrate this centrality well, demonstrating the power of language through the application of questions that lead the person to recognise strengths beyond problem talk. Even slight alterations in sentence construction can make the difference between guiding a person toward problem resolution or the more desirable state of empowering an individual to reach their own unique answers that fit their particular lifestyle, the latter approach raising self-esteem and empowering the person to take control of their life and make their own choices and decisions.

Practice example

A strengths-based approach moves attention away from questions like 'What is the problem?' or 'How can I help you?' towards broader questions that can lead to discovery of a person's own resources to promote change: How have you coped this long? What happens on the days when you manage this problem? What does a good day look like to you?

This subtle change in the language content of questions has the ability to produce significant changes for the person by moving away from discussion of the problem and towards recognising their own strengths, resources and abilities to, if not solve the problem, at least achieve improvements that reduce the impact of the difficulty in their life.

While strengths-based approaches deploy precision language to achieve positive change, the opposite, in the form of careless, ambiguous use of language, can lead to misunderstandings that result in unintended consequences. Examples below illustrate the difficulties that can emerge when there is a lack of consideration about how messages are delivered.

• *The boss said have a great day, so I went home.*

• *Jane took my coat and told me to make myself at home, so I went upstairs for a nap.*

• *The sign said, 'Dogs must be carried on the escalator'. I didn't have one, so I borrowed the neighbour's.*

If we wish our communication to be understood correctly, there is a need to be mindful about its content, particularly when social work communications can have a significant impact on the decisions and actions taken.

Practice example

The note left from the telephone call stated: 'Daisy said she was in a hurry, so she put her daughter in the bath in her pyjamas.'

If Daisy meant she was in her pyjamas because she was late and was washing her child, there would be no concerns; if Daisy was trying to bathe her daughter while her daughter was clothed in pyjamas, then the social worker might have cause for further conversation with Daisy to find out what was happening.

Precision of language is important; often it falls short in communication due to distraction or the presence of other numerous competing factors. A mindful practice can provide a quiet space in the mind in which accurate language can be used to give correct meaning to the messaging that needs to take place. Awareness in the present moment, allowing one to focus on the purpose and content of communication, serves to enhance clarity in this aspect of communication. The quiet, calmer mind that results from mindful practice enables the engagement of micro mindful pauses before speaking or writing in order to connect with awareness of the implications of the message to be given, creating opportunities for clear, concise communication that will be understood.

In short, mindfulness enables the mindful social worker to better curate communications to the benefit of mutual understanding, providing a solid foundation on which to make decisions about actions.

Take-home message

It is easy to misinterpret meaning, and equally to convey confusion. Mindful use of language, which involves stopping and checking meaning while also endeavouring to be precise in the words used, can enhance mutual understanding while avoiding ambiguity that might misdirect towards the pursuit of the wrong goals or actions.

What are you trying to say?

 Verbal communication is further complicated within a professional context by the use of professional language: shorthand communication techniques for those included in the professional circle, but which can be mystifying to outsiders. A technical language often evolves that creates unnecessary communication barriers within and across organisations, but also importantly between social workers and service users. Subsumed within a world of professional abbreviations, social workers can become susceptible to the use of professional language in discussion with service users, rendering them unable to provide explanations in terms the service users will understand. Mindfulness practice offers a means of disrupting these habits and of reconnecting the professional self with the intention of the communication, enabling space for adjustments to be made to ensure its meaning is understood. The need to move away from the habit of using professional language becomes ever more important when it is the underlying obstacle to the accurate representation of the adult's or child's voice in meetings or documentation, as words are converted into technical interpretation by the practitioner without explicit thought about how their meaning might have changed in the process. Mindfulness in the use of language can disrupt this tendency, fostering a more accurate reflection of the views of people receiving services.

There is nothing more isolating as a parent caught up in the child pro-tection system than sitting in a meeting listening to professionals using language or jargon you do not understand.

(Surviving Safeguarding, 2018)

Mindful awareness of the need to adjust conversation to common language that is inclusive, not exclusive, can remedy such deficits. Taking time to notice the terms that we use as professionals and to substitute easily understood phrases to explain services or interventions will lead to flourishing, meaningful conversations that will support partnership collaboration in what is achievable.

Mindful point of reflection

Take a pause to consider the social work role and the field in which you work. Note the different abbreviations or technical words that would not be easily understood by friends or family who do not work in the profession. These are the terms you need to substitute with simpler, easily recognised terms.

Paralanguage

 It is firmly understood that words alone cannot always imply the meaning intended within the message (Thompson, 2020). However, additional means of communication to amplify the intended meaning of contact are available. Present from birth as a necessity for pre-verbal transmission, they remain to enhance understanding; collectively these characteristics are termed paralanguage. They include not only tone, volume and speed of speech, variations of which might indicate states of stress or calm for example, but also other physical gestures or behaviour, collectively termed body language. Often paralanguage can say far more than words alone. A smile might indicate recognition of a person, happiness, shared humour or kindness; it is a universal language for everyone that when appropriate to context can indicate a message that needs no verbal clarification. Equally a communication may appear neutral in its delivery, but if reinforced by a raised voice may provoke alarm or greater attention from the listener: for example, 'Quiet please' can be a calm instruction, but if accompanied by a louder tone indicates a degree of impatience and the requirement for immediate action from an audience. The evolution of virtual communication continues to reflect human endeavours to enhance the meaning of messages with paralanguage. These have emerged through emojis, icons, the use of capitals, bold, highlighting and underlining, to name but a few.

This is a complicated, nuanced area of study, with some additions of tone or gesture being intentional, while others unconsciously emerge, reflecting conflict or internal operations of the mind. Perhaps this is best illustrated by the game of poker, which relies on players recognising small micro-indicators in the opposition's paralanguage as 'tells' that show the internal workings of the player's mind.

The alignment of paralanguage with verbal messaging is an important additional clue for the correct interpretation of communications by the receiver. For a profession such as social work, which is dependent on good communication traits, mastering the skill of alignment is vital not only for effective collaboration with service users and colleagues but also for the implementation of effective safeguarding measures. Clear indicators of tone or body language provide reinforcing signals that ensure a conversation is travelling in its intended direction without misdirection or triggers of confusion that can lead to anger or early termination of a positive interaction. Equally, social workers should be alive to the observation of paralanguage in other people; while verbal messaging might indicate agreement to a course of action, lack of eye contact might raise questions about the level of commitment to the agreed plans, or it might simply be how the person chooses to interact. But the signal, if observed, acts as a cue with which the mindful social worker can explore further for clarification. Noticing these discrepancies helps the social worker to tailor communications within both professional interactions and those with service users. The latter group carries with it greater implications when paralanguage is misinterpreted, as there may be a failure to recognise when an adult or child is experiencing coercion from others in their life, with a subsequent missed safeguarding opportunity.

The application or observation of paralanguage also translates into written communications, where the use of intonation or reinforcement through the script icons on software or via icons in text speak demonstrates the need to extend beyond words to make ourselves understood. Often it is possible to regret the general presentation and content of an email or text sent in anger or speedily without thought. Adopting the practice of taking a mindful pause, facilitating closer attention to the message, its intention and how it will be received, serves to reduce instances of blind reactivity of the mind to contacts that trigger a rapid thoughtless response that can be the cause of harm. These are difficult to repair, remaining as a virtual record that cannot be easily erased.

Practice example

You are about to have a conversation with Bryn about his return home after an operation on a broken hip in hospital. Bryn has recently been diagnosed with dementia and is cared for by his son, who lives with him. Your discussion will involve finding out how best to support Bryn in his care. Identify the paralanguage signs that might come from Bryn and his son as you try to understand what is working and not working, and what a good day looks like.

The full picture

Context adds a further layer that needs to be considered when trying to communicate effectively, particularly when reading the 'mood in the room'; this cannot be achieved if, while we are physically present, our minds are elsewhere, either in a previous meeting or contact or anticipating the next action beyond the present encounter. The skill of contextual communication relies on our full arrival in the present moment, our giving attention to the surroundings and the demeanour of those we are interacting with, and the establishment of objective perceptions of events as they arise. Taking mindful opportunities to pause, breathe and wait for emotions or reactions from a previous meeting or visit to dissipate before launching into the next engagement mitigates habitual reactivity, allowing the mind to be calm, creating space for greater awareness of what is happening and what might be appropriate within the context of communication of the moment.

Practice example

Examples in which contextual awareness matters for good communication:

- *being fully present to the depth of grief a person might be experiencing at a sudden loss, enabling the social worker to adapt their manner and conversation to the level of sadness in the meeting;*

- *exhibiting greater awareness of a person's anxiety at the presence of others in the household, prompting a social work response to seek a conversation, perhaps in a different context to the home, to enable the person to speak freely;*

- *noticing a tense atmosphere in the home while people are endeavouring to present a happy picture, allowing social work observation to reveal the tension and to explore its origins and resolution, or to reflect on the need, perhaps, for a safeguarding response, both of which involve adapting the course of action to the context of the meeting.*

The value of contextual awareness extends to the observation of cultural customs and norms and their place in interactions. It is not expected that social workers should have expert knowledge of all the customs and cultural traditions that are present within a multicultural society. However, approaching encounters with mindful openness, responding to the context with insightful co-operation that respects others' cultural traditions and balancing these alongside the purpose of the social work intervention, whether it be safeguarding or support, requires sensitive communication guided by objective perception. Mindful practice that builds a breadth of awareness with a quietened mind enhances one's ability to step back from situations to observe what is actually taking place and to adapt communication, behaviour and language to the cultural context, responding to cultural cues provided by those present. This strength ensures communication is situationally appropriate, serving to support the objective outcome of intervention, without causing offence or mistrust in a relationship.

Take-home message

A mindful approach can marry aspects of communication in harmony to meet the situation as it presents, helping social workers to curate self with clear, intended messages.

Listening

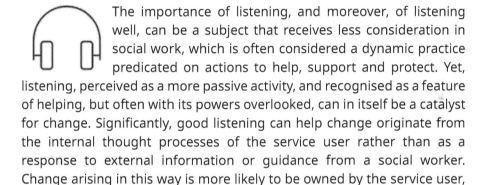

The importance of listening, and moreover, of listening well, can be a subject that receives less consideration in social work, which is often considered a dynamic practice predicated on actions to help, support and protect. Yet, listening, perceived as a more passive activity, and recognised as a feature of helping, but often with its powers overlooked, can in itself be a catalyst for change. Significantly, good listening can help change originate from the internal thought processes of the service user rather than as a response to external information or guidance from a social worker. Change arising in this way is more likely to be owned by the service user, resulting in their greater commitment to following it through to success.

> *Like so many of us I used to take listening for granted, glossing over this step as I rushed into more active, visible ways of being helpful. Now, I am convinced that listening is the single most important element of any helpful relationship. Listening has great power. It draws thoughts and feelings out of people as nothing else can.*
>
> *When someone listens to you well, you become more aware of feelings you may not have realized you felt. You have ideas you may have never thought before.*
>
> (Lipman, 1998)

Listening well is not a skill that features prominently as part of social work training, yet it has the capacity to enhance a person's value and self-esteem and to empower them to process information and work out their own solutions to difficulties; it leads to greater understanding, creating more informed, appropriate forms of social work intervention.

Practice example

Note the difference between conversations A and B. Which one demonstrates listening well and provides the clearer basis for beneficial social work intervention?

Conversation A

Social worker	Are you a single parent?
Mother:	Yes, my partner died, but I have...
SW:	So, you look after the children alone?
Mother:	Yes.
SW:	Can you take them to school on time then, as there have been concerns?
Mother:	I do, but Charlotte is often late in the mornings because...
SW:	Perhaps a taxi might help?
Mother:	Yes, that would be good but...
SW:	Good. I will put that in place, and we will have no more late attendance.

Conversation B

SW:	Are you a single parent?
Mother:	Yes, my partner died but I have my mother to help.
SW:	So you look after the children alone?
Mother:	I do. I am worried as Charlotte is often late to school in the mornings.
SW:	Why is that happening do you think? Take your time.

Mother:	Well, she doesn't sleep well since David died in his accident. In fact, none of us do.
SW:	I'm sorry that must be very difficult.
Mother:	I think if I have someone to talk to about it and some advice about how to deal with the children's grief it might help.
SW:	I will investigate the kinds of help that might be available as a starting point. Do you think a conversation with the school in the meantime to find out how best they can support you and Charlotte might help?
Mother:	Yes, that might be a way forward.
SW:	Would you like any support from anyone with that conversation? Perhaps your mother, or myself?
Mother:	I think my mum can help with those, thanks.
SW:	I will call back next week with an update. If you think of anything else in the meantime, write it down and we can talk it through on our next meeting. Do you have my contact details?
Mother	Yes, thanks.

Listening well

Listening well begins with the creation of a time and space in which a person can talk or communicate their narrative at their pace, in a comfortable, safe environment. Mindfully approaching the arrangement of conversational environments that are conducive to the sharing of what can be difficult, sensitive information is a crucial enabler of open and honest communication that can lead to greater insight into the nature of social work help. Consideration should be given to the time of meeting, whether it is convenient, and whether there will be other pressing matters at that point in the day (for example, children returning home from school, medical visits to an older person in a care home). Paying mindful attention to the meeting venue, particularly its possible meaning for the service user is also important. For instance, is school a good place to talk with a child about their difficulties at home when it is the only place they feel able to forget about them? Or is it just convenient for the professional because the child is there and can be withdrawn easily from lessons to come and talk? Equally, is the older person interviewed in a care home inhibited because they feel people are listening to the conversation?

Mindful point of reflection

Consider what might make a comfortable time and place for you to have a conversation about something that is important to you. What are the factors that influence this decision? Consider the same factors in relation to people you work with: what might support or impede conversations? This reflection can help to provide mindful insight into planning to listen well.

Listening well necessitates being quiet, an action that can be counterintuitive to social work, which is driven by verbal advice and helpfulness. Being quiet leads to a silence that the other person can inhabit to convey their story and intended meaning. Taylor (2015) ponders if there is too much talk in social work, highlighting mindfulness as a means to promote the use of silence as a contemplative tool to achieve reflection in practice. Mindful meditation, taking time out or opportunities during the day to pause and focus quietly on the breath, enables the social work practitioner to become comfortable with silence, a characteristic that transfers into everyday life and which has value when listening to others. The maintaining of silence gives time to the person talking to communicate their thoughts, feelings and emotions effectively, and it allows a moment for the person to digest information and formulate an accurate response. But most of all, silence, accompanied by attentive listening, reflects an atmosphere that empowers the other person, respecting their views or opinions and providing an invitation to collaborate about the next steps in a plan of action. All of this contributes to a greater understanding that informs intelligent responses and actions.

The difference between hearing and listening

The difference between hearing and listening is attention, interrupting sound with focused attention to what is being said or communicated. Kadushin and Kadushin (1997) differentiate the two by highlighting hearing as a physical act and listening as a cerebral one predicated on understanding. Mindfulness enhances development of the latter trait: its practice of paying attention to the breath and noticing but not responding to distracting thoughts provides discipline to the meditator, facilitating the development of skills that remain after the completion of meditation itself. In a social work setting, such skills are invaluable for self-management, providing resistance against the urge to interrupt or dominate conversations with helpful guidance and assisting the social worker to listen with curiosity to messages being given. Such attentiveness prompts intuitive questions and the noticing of paralanguage, often termed 'listening with the third ear', and the ability to see the gaps in language, what is not said, where sensitive questions might be needed in order to pursue further. The power of mindfulness to reduce the traffic of the mind, alongside the control to not interact with thoughts as they arise, guards against distraction or mind-wandering when listening as part of the social work role, which demonstrates respect to the communicator while also ensuring the best circumstances for complete understanding. Concentration of this nature facilitates opportunities to reflect understanding back to the other person or to use feedback techniques to gain greater clarification of particular points. It helps us avoid the need to request repetition or to risk showing the communicator they did not have our full attention, something that might discourage dialogue in future or risk trust in the relationship.

Take-home message

It is important to be vigilant against mind-wandering and to listen well. It is not enough to merely hear the words someone is saying, it is also important to bring attention to the whole communication in order to fully understand.

Understanding and being understood are the foundations for success in social work practice. Neither are simple tasks, and anything that might help to make them easier should be welcomed. While communication skills can be talked about, illustrated or highlighted as an important aspect of social work training, mindfulness is a key concept that can provide genuine changes in the brain that support this most basic of instincts. Social workers who aspire to clarity in communication and the ability to utilise it to create sustainable change that arises within the individual rather than from professional external pressure, no matter how gentle, would be advised to include mindfulness in the practice toolkit. Just a few minutes of focused attention on the breath, regularly, as part of a daily routine, can change our communication functionality for the better.

Takeaways

1. Key points

- Good communication is the key to good social work.

- Communication is reciprocal: it includes both talking and listening.

- The power of listening as an activity of change by itself is not always recognised within the helping professions. Providing a sounding board for a person to process their own thoughts, feelings and emotions before deciding on a chosen course of action can at times be all that is needed. This simple yet effective method of support needs more attention.

- Mindfulness changes the brain in a way that enhances our ability to communicate, to connect with people around us. Increased attention, a quieter mind and the use of present awareness free from distractions enhance the quality of our engagement with others.

- The more we talk, the less we understand in social work. Mindful use of silence creates space for a person to inhabit and share their story, helping us understand what is significant to them. Our responses and support become more intelligent as a result.

2. Straight talking: Letting go of the jargon. Here are some examples

Abuse	Harm caused by someone who has power over the victim.
Assessment	The process of working out what is needed: gathering information, facts and opinions, making judgements, agreeing what is most important and figuring out what kind of support might help.

Outcomes	Things a person wants to happen in their life.
Prevention	Support and help to stop small problems getting bigger.
Referral	Request for a service from an organisation.
Consent	Agreement given to care and support.
Informed consent	Having all the information necessary to make a decision to agree

3. Working with distraction

Listening and responding well depend upon focused, unswerving attention to what is happening in the moment of communication. Distraction inevitably occurs, but the stronger we are at resisting it, whether it is in our own thoughts or external in the environment, the better our communication will be. Mindful meditation on the breath, noticing thoughts as they arise without engaging, and returning to the breath when it is noticed that we have strayed, will build skill in concentration. The practice of mindful meditation when walking will reinforce the mind's ability to resist distraction further. The resources in the Resource hut at the end of this book will point you in the direction of places where guidance about walking meditation can be found. However, it can be as simple as the steps outlined below:

Walking meditation

 Walking unhurriedly, breathe in and out slowly, focusing on the breath. Notice your feet touching the ground, the sounds and sights as you move along. Feel any wind, rain or sun on your face and body. Eventually, your breathing will attune to the rhythm of your feet, relaxation will arrive in your body, distracting thoughts will subside. Regular mindful walking will help to increase concentration on the topics you choose rather than on those that present themselves, the latter of which lead to the mind wandering off the subject at hand.

4. Touching base with the present

Create a reminder to fully arrive in the present, casting off any previous emotions, thoughts or information from the previous meeting, visit or encounter. Identify a space in the office or car where you will touch base with yourself through mindfulness before moving on to your next thing.

5. Seeking feedback

Engage with trusted friends or family to tell you how well you communicate or listen. This will give indicators of where you might need to focus mindful awareness in order to make improvements.

6. Mindful micro-moment tip

Taking the opportunity to build mindful micro-moments for pause and reflection can enable the mindful social worker to recognise times when a reset is needed in communication in order to put it on the right track.

References and further reading

Cupack, B, Spitberg, H and William, R (1994) *The Dark Side of Interpersonal Communication*. New York: Routledge.

Dickson, D and Bamford, D (1995) Improving the Inter-Personal Skills of Social Work Students: The Problem of Transfer Learning and What to Do About It. *British Journal of Social Work*, 25(1): 85–105.

Hopkins, G (1998) *Plain English for Social Services: A Guide for Better Communication*. Lyme Regis: Russell House.

Kadushin, A and Kadushin, G (1997) *The Social Work Interview*, 4th edition. New York: Columbia University Press.

Lipman, D (1998) *The Storytelling Coach: How to Listen, Praise and Bring Out People's Best*. Little Rock Arizona: August House.

Lishman, J (2009) *Communication in Social Work*. Basingstoke: Macmillan/ BASW.

Nelsen, J (1980) *Communication Theory and Social Work Practice*. Chicago: University Chicago Press.

Prince, K (1996) *Boring Records? Communication, Speech and Writing in Social Care and Related Services*. Lyme Regis: Russell House.

Robinson, M (2002) *Communication and Health in a Multi-Ethnic Society*. Bristol: Policy Press.

Surviving Safeguarding (2018) Divisive, Demeaning and Devoid of Feeling: How Social Work Jargon Causes Problems for Families. *Community Care*. [online] Available at: www.communitycare.co.uk/2018/05/10/divisive-demeaning-devoid-feeling-social-work-jargon-causes-problems-families/ (accessed 18 August 2022).

Taylor, R (2015) Do We Talk Too Much in Social Work? *Community Care*. [online] Available at: www.communitycare.co.uk/2015/07/23/talk-much-social-work/ (accessed 18 August 2022).

Thompson, N (1997) Interpersonal Skills-Social Work Module. *New Technology in the Human Services*, 10(2): 21–2.

Thompson, N (2003) *Communication and Language: A Handbook of Theory and Practice*. Basingstoke: Palgrave Macmillan

Thompson, N (2020) *Understanding Social Work: Preparing for Practice*, 5th edition. London: Palgrave.

Thompson, N (2021) *People Skills: A Guide to Effective Practice in the Human Services*, 5th edition. Basingstoke: Palgrave.

Trevithick, P (2012) *Social Work Skills: A Practice Handbook*, 3rd edition. Buckingham: Open University Press.

Chapter 4

Developing trusted relationships

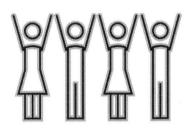

You can't buy trust in the supermarket.

(Dalai Lama)

The ability to develop trusted relationships between social worker and service user, among colleagues and across professional boundaries has always made a valuable contribution to the achievement of positive change for people in their lives. It is only well-balanced, open and honest relationships that enable social work to transcend the superficial, to understand what is going on below the surface for children and adults. Partnerships form the basis for good support to nurture strengths-based approaches for people who use services; partnerships enhanced with trust can make the difference between success or failure in the provision of the right support at the right time.

This chapter will include:

Social work as a relationship-based practice

Leap of faith

Competence

Steering a steady ship

The emotional web

Integrity

Cultural humility

Benevolence

Social work as a relationship-based practice

Social work is firmly rooted in relationship-based practice. This remains the case even during the current growth of managerial social work drivers that enable procedure-driven social work, placing emphasis on perform-ance alongside measurable outcomes. A profession predicated on human relations by necessity holds relationships at its heart (Trevithick, 2003; Alexander and Grant, 2009; O'Leary et al, 2013). Many academic social work commentators have observed that relationships are not merely conduits for intervention but are the intervention itself (Fewster, 2004). One school of thought extends this view further, concluding that any intervention model is demonstrably secondary to the effect of the quality of the relation-ship between service user and social worker (Nicholson and Artze, 2003). Relationships become the most essential element of caring professional practice, acting in themselves as a catalyst for change. *'The relationship is where most of the important things happen, for good or for ill, whether social workers recognise it or not'* (Howe, 1998).

The success of strengths-based models of practice, based on cultur-ally sensitive interactions, is dependent on the emergence of trusting relationships between practitioner and service user, alongside pro-fessional disciplinary connections. Trust becomes the transformative element of social work relationships; proficiency in the development of trust becomes central to the role.

Mindfulness can be drawn upon to aid the social worker in this develop-ment by enabling the mindful social worker to personify trust, demon-strating behaviour, qualities and actions that encourage people to place their trust in the social work relationship. *'Mindfulness facilitates a person's ability to engage in behaviours that create trusting relationships'* (Steadham and Skaar, 2019, p 1).

Steadham and Skaar (2019) use an organisational model of trust (Mayer et al, 1995) to demonstrate the contribution mindfulness can make to the development of employees' trust in leadership. These same principles are applied in this chapter to illustrate how mindfulness can contribute to the presence of trust in a service user/social work relationship, nested within a trusting professional network that facilitates a cohesive, multi-partner approach to intervention.

Leap of faith

 Trust can be defined as a leap of faith or 'trust leap' that involves a person who is vulnerable and uncertain placing confidence in the good intentions or actions of another. It can be defined as *'a psychological state comprising the intention to accept vulnerability based upon the positive expectations of the intentions or behaviour of another'* (Rousseau et al, 1998). In the case of social work, the service user or fellow professional places confidence in the social worker, making a connection that forms a trusted relationship.

The formation of trust can be encouraged by three essential identifying features that reduce vulnerability or uncertainty on the part of the trustor (service user or professional) in relation to the trustee (social worker), increasing the likelihood of trust in the relationship: competence, integrity and benevolence (Mayer et al, 1995). Adaptation of the conceptual framework proposed by Steadman and Skaar illustrates the contribution mindfulness can make to the presence of trust in the often complex, mistrustful arena of social work practice.

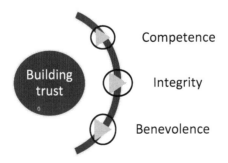

Figure 4.1 Three key elements of building trust

Take-home message

Trust is the vital ingredient at the heart of social work practice needed for relationships to work. It requires a leap of faith by those using services, and social workers must work hard to reassure service users that the leap is well founded.

Competence

The presence of competence is apparent if it is evident that the social worker has the skills, knowledge and capability to meet the demands of the role. Both service users and colleagues alike will place trust in the relationship if they can identify the social worker as competent, reassuring the trustor of the likelihood of positive outcomes and reducing feelings of uncertainty.

Competence in social work is increased through knowledge, skill and experience. But building trust through competency is also dependent on how these qualities are deployed in practice. The application of a set model of practice, a one-size-fits-all approach, will only carry social work practice so far; although there are often commonalities across presenting situations, there are often surprises unique to the service user within each individual interaction.

If the social worker is wrong-footed, or unable to adapt to the situation as it is rather as they expect it to be, competence is lost along with the trust of the service user as uncertainty and anxiety emerge.

Working with reality not expectation

The mindful quality of present awareness, which discards habitual reactivity, acts as an antidote to social work practice that operates from a point of expectation based on previous social work experience, changing the practice into one that works with the reality of the situation. This creates space for the social work practitioner to draw appropriately on knowledge, skill and experience to meet the needs of each service user anew, recognising their expertise and negotiating a trusting partnership approach that moves beyond a fixed model of application. The perception shifts that can arise from mindfulness create opportunities for the mindful social worker to see the issues from the other person's viewpoint. This supports a relationship based on negotiation and partnership in pursuit of solutions, reducing anxiety on the part of the person receiving services. Space is created in which the social worker can demonstrate competency in an adaptive, responsive approach to meet the person's unique needs while also fostering the formation of trust in the relationship, which can become the bedrock of positive change.

Practice example

Sil is visiting Frank as part of a safeguarding response. Frank is an 81-year-old man who has started to have a personal relationship with his cleaner, May. Frank's son is worried that May is exploiting Frank for money, Frank has recently bought her a new car.

The encounter between Sil and Frank does not go well. Sil has personal experience of older people being exploited for money, as something similar happened to his grandfather. He is very angry at the thought of such scams, and is clear with Frank that there is a risk of financial harm. Sil describes how these scams work and advises Frank he should end the relationship for his own safety. Sil also lets Frank know that he will ask Frank's son to keep an eye on him. Frank becomes very angry, asks Sil to leave and tells him that social workers should never contact him again, no matter what the circumstances are.

Reflect on how Sil could have handled the situation differently to create trust with Frank.

Steering a steady ship

Self-control and emotional regulation both need to be evi-dent qualities in any competent social worker, it is of no help to a service user whose life might be falling apart for the social worker to fall apart with them, a situation which would inspire neither confidence nor trust in the person who needs help.

Mindfulness is central to the maintenance of these qualities, providing the practitioner with 'seer' abilities of self-observation to regulate thoughts and emotional reactions and to maintain objectivity in difficult predicaments. The mindful approach of observing one's own thoughts objectively, without engaging in emotional reactivity, leads to the professional skill of observation without emotional baggage and the reduction of those emotive, irrational responses that likely lead to service user mistrust. The absence of emotional entanglement in social work professional practice creates mental space for an increase in cognitive capacity and flexibility (Shapiro et al, 2005), which enables the social worker to demonstrate competence in action.

The emotional web

The propensity of the mindful social worker to objectively engage with relationships, enjoying increased cognition with adaptive abilities, becomes a valuable commodity in social work relationships which uncover difficult interactions that need to be handled skilfully. The presence of transference and counter-transference in relations is a case in point.

Transference and counter-transference refer to the unconscious application of past experiences, particularly those of being parented, to the formation and maintenance of current relationships. Recognition of the behaviours linked to early childhood relationships, particularly in relation to parental or primary caregiver experiences, give important clues to the way in which relationships are managed as adults.

Practice example

An example of this kind of transference is when we identify someone as a 'people pleaser', someone seeking praise or endorsement that had not been provided by parents or carers during their early years. A social worker may encounter the person as someone who readily agrees or complies, but a dependency is created that leads to an inability to sustain positive change when the social work intervention ends.

Ruch et al (2010) highlight the service user's transference of past negative experiences of parenting into a current relationship with a social
worker, in which the social worker may unwittingly start to experience
the anger, sadness or fear of the service user, without realisation that
projection of the person's feelings is taking place. Counter-transference
can also occur, whereby the social worker may react unconsciously from
past experience, completing the transference/counter-transference cycle
(Figure 4.2). Enactment of the cycle is unlikely to lead to a successful, positive conclusion.

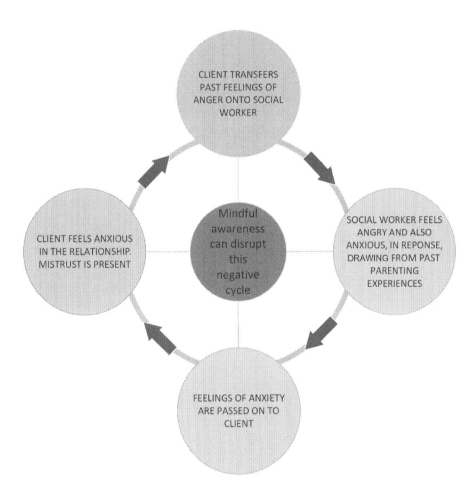

Figure 4.2 Transference/counter-transference cycle

Present awareness through mindfulness provides opportunity for the mindful social worker to recognise when something as complex as transference is taking place, allowing the social worker to marshal responses that disrupt the transference cycle, shifting the relationship onto safer ground where trust can be built. Skilled self-management in these situations demonstrates competency in the role that amplifies trust within the service user/social work relationship, as well as in those professionals who observe the capabilities of the social worker as 'self in action' (Ingram and Smith, 2018).

Trust in self

Competence can be amplified through the mindful social work embodiment of trust itself. Mindful meditation provides the means to connect with trust in self through personal understanding. *'In practicing mindfulness, you are taking responsibility for being yourself and learning to listen to and trust your own being'* (Kabat-Zinn, nd). The development of trust in self enhances confidence within practice, providing clarity of judgement. The resultant reduction of professional insecurity creates a practice of transparency, one open to challenges and in which there is a willingness to consider other perspectives. Combined, these traits provide reassurance of the authenticity of the social worker, while also building professional resilience in the face of negative challenges.

This becomes apparent in the management of conflict, which inevitably emerges in the social work arena, both with service users, as a result of limited resources or the imposition of actions that are not welcome, or across professional relationships in areas of pressure or blame. Conflict that is handled well can be productive as a catalyst for the development of trust; if responded to poorly it can result in the harmful severance of relationships. Increased competence along with emotional regularity, mental space and the ability to focus on the present equip the mindful social worker with traits to assist good conflict management and resolution. The propensity to resist reactivity permits a timely pause in order to evaluate the wisest course of action in response to conflictual situations. Resilience created through competency gives way to a response of compassion, one involving patience rather than anger and which is more likely to result in early resolution of differences, with increased capacity for trust. This becomes a particularly important skill for working with service users (both adults and children) who may have felt let down by people in the past or experienced broken trust, but who use conflict as a means of testing the professional relationship. Responses that are calm and compassionate demonstrate consistent dependability that helps to give reassurance of the mindful social worker's reliability.

These positive developments, which are consequences of mindful practice, elicit a presentation of professional consistency: predictable, reliable behaviour that encourages the service user to put their faith in the social work relationship.

Mindful point of reflection

Bring to mind an example of social work practice or intervention that you have undertaken. Focus on how you used self in the practice: What attitudes and behaviours did you demonstrate? Where did they come from? What worked well? And what needs to change?

Integrity

Social workers who act with professional integrity encourage service users' trust in the relationship. Mayer et al (1995) observed that trustors were more likely to place trust in a trustee if they perceived the trustee adhering to a set of principles or values that governed their actions, particularly if the trustor agreed with the principles in place. In social work terms, this facilitates service users' or colleagues' recognition that the social worker is operating within a professional framework that guides actions or decisions, limiting the occurrence of random, unpredictable events that might be perceived as threatening. A shared understanding or agreement regarding the rules of operation further enhances the stability of the social work relationship, encouraging trust through partnership.

Social work, as a self-in-action profession, has an explicit framework of values, principles and attitudes that govern practice. This requires the social worker to curate their personal lifeview alongside professional requirements; self-knowledge is essential to the achievement of this goal. Without self-knowledge, social work becomes blind habitual reaction based on values or principles obtained through past experience where there has been no change or development. The interplay between personal and professional beliefs, attitudes, values and experiences provides the foundation of such cycles of response. In order to build trust, social workers will need to surface these elements both personally and professionally, and be able to apply them intelligently in a way that demonstrates integrity of practice. The objectivity and self-observation skills that are developed through mindful practice can serve to enhance abilities in these areas of the personality.

Self-knowledge

The role of the social worker as 'self in action' brings into sharp focus the importance of self-knowledge in supporting effective practice. Self is the point of most control, influencing behaviours and attitudes that reflect trust. Looking within provides increased understanding of personhood in relation to personal and professional identity, allowing the mindful social worker to reconcile both in the demonstration of a practice governed by an explicit, value-based professional framework

A focus on internal insight yields information that helps to manage emotions, feelings, actions and behaviour in a way that garners trust as a foundation for relationship-based practice. Developing an understanding of the personal narrative helps to enhance awareness of mind and personality functioning, enabling empathetic action to take place, an essential ingredient for a trusting relationship. Engagement with people whose experiences make it difficult to trust requires patience, empathy and understanding. Recognising these personal traits through mindful practice enhances one's competence to apply them appropriately in a professional setting.

Putting the mind house in order

 Everyone has their own unique personal narrative shaped by individual experiences, culture, spiritual beliefs and environment. It is the prism through which each person engages with the world, governing responses to all that is encountered. Much of one's personal narrative has been formed through early childhood, influenced by family, friends or education and reinforced or questioned depending on one's personal experience in the world. It is the foundation of who we are, and when challenged it can evoke defensive responses as if we feel that our very core is under threat.

Beliefs	Values	Attitudes
Ideas that you hold to be true. They can arise out of your own direct experience, through societal or cultural norms, from information you read or hear or from a trusted person you regard as creditable.	Values form out of beliefs that you hold to be true. They become a guide for how you form opinions, react to situations and make decisions.	Beliefs and values shape your attitudes to situations in life and also shape your responses. They influence your attitudes to relationships both personal and professional.
Examples:	*Examples:*	*Examples:*
You should do your best at work. People should not break the law. People should not be judged by their appearance.	Honesty is the best policy. Respect people's privacy. Show kindness to people. Treat people equally.	Distrusting a colleague you believe to be untruthful. Mistrusting someone who you feel is favouring their friends with services rather than treating everyone equally.

But here's the thing

 Life is subject to continual change: beliefs and values might not always be founded on solid ground; some may be incompatible with the professional framework of social work, others may inhibit the productive formation of trusted relationships with both professional colleagues and service users. Problems occur when there is a reluctance to let go of an established narrative, particularly when it is reinforced by contact solely with others of similar beliefs and without experience of different perspectives. Often professional decisions can be made not in relation to an external professional framework that is clear to everyone involved but based on the internal narrative that is often not consciously acknowledged by the social worker, in whom it manifests as merely a habitual response based on an established view of the world. In this habitual state, the formation of trust is inhibited, as those who encounter social work practice are unable to easily discern the professional basis of decisions that might on the face of it appear unjust or irrational. Without explicit demonstration of decisions or actions within professional standards, those who need to trust social workers are unable to have confidence in the integrity of the professional before them.

The mindful process of getting to know self by drawing internal beliefs, values and attitude to the forefront of the mind and considering them with questioning curiosity becomes an invaluable first step towards ensuring the professional governance of social work practice, serving to counteract subconscious, automatic action based on past personal experiences and influences which may introduce unconscious bias into the equation and serve as fertile ground only for mistrust.

Practice example

Consider the questions below and provide your answers. What might you need to adapt and change in order to build trust with others?

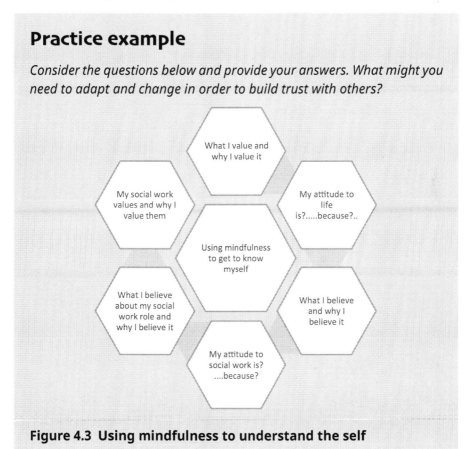

Figure 4.3 Using mindfulness to understand the self

Mindful meditation promotes self-inquiry, leading to self-awareness, which Parker et al (2015) describe as intrapersonal awareness of internal attunement between the observing and the experiencing self. The increase in self-awareness, translated into social work practice, enables the mindful social worker to make considered choices that align with the external, professional value framework rather than the personal, reactive formations. Once the social work professional's value base is explicitly established as the compass for practice, a reduction in reactivity occurs, with an increase in emotional regulation. Service users and colleagues alike are able to perceive a social worker who is referencing a clear professional framework that supports consistency in rational actions, and this in turn provides assurances that the social worker is a trustworthy professional, providing the added advantage of helping to balance the inevitable power differentials between social worker and service user. A shared agreement about the explicit standards guiding social work actions serves to redress the inequality that occurs as a result of the social worker's being seen as a gatekeeper of resources or imposer of sanctions. It places permission or consent with the service user while also providing them with measures for complaint if it is felt that there is an abuse of power. *'Social workers should work in a way that is honest, reliable and open. Clearly explain role, interventions and decisions'* (BASW, 2021).

Self-awareness regarding the interplay between the personal and professional value realms enhances the social worker's ability to recognise when bias may be infringing or inhibiting the implementation of professional decision-making. The mindful social worker is better able to restrict the human tendency to rush to judgement on the basis of internal, unacknowledged private beliefs or experiences, and is able to observe the situation as it presents in actuality rather than providing an interpretation through private life filters. This models professional integrity through the ensuing opportunities it creates for trust to be built on neutral territory.

Practice example

Mindful reflective exercise

Read the information in the case below. Place to one side the content and the automatic reaching of the mind for actions or solutions, but notice in the first instance the feelings and reactions that arise for you. What judgements do you make? What beliefs or standards are you applying to this scenario? Mindfully observe your responses and notice what is instinctive and what you can attribute to your own personal narrative interpretation.

The case of MM

MM is a female adult living with paranoid schizophrenia. Prominent visual, auditory and tactile hallucinations were significant features for MM of the mental health condition. MM also had moderate learning disabilities and appeared unable to demonstrate insight into her health needs. Now an adult, she had grown up in care following chaotic and emotionally absent experiences of being parented. She met her partner K at a homeless hostel, and they had already been in a relationship for 15 years. K also had mental health needs with a psychopathic personality. He abused alcohol and lived a transient lifestyle that included MM. It is believed that K had also been physically violent to MM. During periods of homelessness MM had not taken her medication, leading to a deterioration in her mental health.

The local authority were seeking to make MM safe and felt that they needed to take control of decisions about where MM should live, with whom she could associate and management of finances. They sought to protect MM, and believed she lacked mental capacity to make these decisions herself.

(Local Authority X v MM & Anor, 2007)

Find the place in your response where professional values and standards are triggered.

Cultural humility

It is not necessary to have expert knowledge of variations in culture, and indeed it would be impossible, since even within different recognisable cultures, variations about how cultural norms are applied exist. What is important, in order to demonstrate one's competence as a trustworthy professional, is to be mindful that culture exists, to have mindful curiosity about people's culture and how it impacts the social service intervention taking place. Barsky (2018) uses the apt term *'cultural humility'*: acknowledging that we do not know everything about a person's culture and using reflection and self-awareness to nurture our cultural sensitivity, while also bringing into play our mindful curiosity about the culture adopted by the person we are working with. This does not mean withdrawing from necessary social work actions such as safeguarding, but rather means delivering the services in a culturally sensitive way. *'Social Workers don't need to be highly knowledgeable about different cultures, but must be open, respectful and willing to learn'* (Hardy, 2018).

Holding cultural humility mindfully at the forefront of practice enables the mindful social worker to embrace diversity, thus developing a broader line of sight to the world that opens up discussions with those who access services. Shifting away from established assumptions about culture and towards mindful curiosity about difference facilitates intercultural compe-tence, through which lies a path to shared solutions in which the service user becomes a true partner in the journey. *'It is not our differences that divide us. It is our inability to recognise, accept and celebrate those differences'* (Audre Lorde Quotes, nd).

Cultural humility places the mindful social worker not in a position of weakness but in one of strength through integrity and competence. Pursuit of mindful curiosity regarding difference opens up a world of pre-viously unseen possibilities in social work practice. This lifelong approach of self-awareness through mindfulness enables the mindful social worker to meet the service user where they are, not where a social worker thinks they should be, a step that promotes trust in the relationship.

Mindful point of reflection

What assumptions do you hold about different cultures? What are they based on? What questions could you ask to demonstrate cultural humility in these instances?

 ## Take-home message

Social workers can use mindful self-insight to embody the values and standards of their professional compass.

Benevolence

Benevolence is the third essential component of trust (Mayer et al, 1995); trustors need to believe that the trustee is operating with their best interests in mind. This can manifest itself in the perception of the social worker as a caring individual who keeps the service user's needs and well-being at the centre of practice. Here too, mindfulness can make its contribution .

> *People high in dispositional mindfulness and experienced mindfulness meditators are often described as warm people, humans who are intimately in touch with the joys and sufferings of their fellow humans*
> (Parker et al, 2015)

Meditation focuses on the observation of thoughts rather than engagement with them, treating them without judgement but with kindness and compassion to self, predisposing the mindful social worker to align with the internal state of another, recognising when compassion or kindness is needed.

Scientific study has identified the changes that meditation can make to the elements of the brain associated with empathetic response. Bernhardt and Singer (2012) identified the anterior insular and angulate cortex as the regions of the brain that foster empathy. Studies that examined the impact meditation makes on brain formulation have found that the areas of the brain most impacted by meditation included the anterior insula and angulate cortex (Fox et al, 2014).

Furthermore, research that included participants who undertook brief meditation practice alongside participants who were merely distracted found that those who underwent the meditation practice were better able to identify the correct emotional states displayed in photographic facial imaging (Tan et al, 2014).

Mindful activity focusing on self, the inner world, leads to the mindful social worker developing self-empathy awareness that translates into wider empathetic connections outside the meditation practice, increasing emotional intelligence which facilities better recognition of the emotional states of others and providing opportunity for the appropriate expression of empathy. The benevolence manifested builds trust as the service user is reassured that the social worker has their best interests in mind.

Take-home message

Kindness and compassion to self in mindful meditation has the off-cushion benefit of encouraging empathetic responses to others.

Practice example

Applying the mindful trust model – competence, integrity and benevolence

Consider the following case scenario and look for ways that you might promote trust in Pearl and her son, applying the trust model of competence, integrity and benevolence.

Pearl arrived in England from Nigeria six months ago. She is accompanied by her son Chad, who is seven years old. Pearl is living with epilepsy, and health support staff are not certain but think she may have some learning difficulties. Chad attends the local school but is falling behind the other members of his class. He does communicate very well, overcoming any language difficulties. The school reports that Chad is often missing from class. They believe he is looking after his mother; he is often needed to translate for health appointments. Recently, Chad had to call an ambulance for Pearl as she had become unconscious during an epileptic episode. Both Pearl and Chad are very wary of talking to professionals, and it is difficult to meet with them to have a conversation about any help they might need.

Trust is the magic component of relationship-based practice: if it is not present, little can succeed. Holding trust in mind helps to maintain awareness of the impact of the social work self in action and allows one notice whether actions are building a trusting relationship or a destabilising one.

Mindfulness exists as a mechanism that social workers can access to build trust through competence, integrity and benevolence. '*Social workers have a responsibility to respect and uphold the values and principles of the profession and act in a reliable, honest and trustworthy manner*' (BASW, 2021). Pursuit of self-awareness through mindfulness and the maintaining of a mindful reflective practice gives the mindful social worker authenticity, which reassures any person accessing services that their trust in the professional will not be misplaced.

Takeaways

1. Key points

- Relationship-based practice remains at the heart of social work, but there also needs to be the presence of trust to create meaningful relationships.

- Trust is a leap of faith by a person who is vulnerable into the unknown; it requires reassurance from the person who wishes to create the trust.

- Competence, integrity and benevolence are the key elements that support a trust model.

- The mindful practice delivers the qualities that demonstrate competency in a role.

- Self-awareness and reflection through mindfulness help the mindful social worker operate according to their professional compass, promoting integrity of position.

- Self-compassion and kindness during mindful meditation translates into daily social work life through the application of benevolence in practice, reassuring service users that they their best interests are always held in view.

2. Principles and values of social work

Value	Principles
Social work is based on inherent worth and dignity of all people	Upholding and promoting human dignity and well-being
	Respecting the right to self-determination
	Promoting the right to participation
	Working holistically
	Identifying and developing strengths
It is a duty of social work to promote social justice in society in general and with individuals	Challenging oppression
	Respecting diversity
	Distributing resources
	Challenging unjust policies and practices
	Working in solidarity towards an inclusive society
Social workers have a responsibility to respect and uphold the values and principles of the profession and act in a reliable, honest and trustworthy manner	Upholding the values and reputation of the profession
	Working in a way that is honest, reliable and open,
	Clearly explaining roles, interventions and decisions
	Maintaining professional boundaries
	Making considered professional judgements
	Being transparent and professionally accountable.

(The code of ethics for social work, BASW, 2021)

3. Model for a positive relationship between mindfulness and trust

Mindful mechanisms	Social work qualities	Trust	Outcome
Attention Re-perceiving Cognitive capacity Self-regulation of emotions Self-regulation of behaviour Self-awareness Social awareness	Consideration of different explanations Clarity of role and purpose Emotional objectivity Balance of personal and professional value bases Accountability Holding a wider view of profes-sional power balance	Competence Integrity Benevolence	Social work relationship-based practice that embodies trust at its core

(Adapted from Steadham and Skaar's (2019) proposed conceptual frame-work relating mindfulness to leadership effectiveness)

References and further reading

Alexander, C and Grant, C (2009) Caring, Mutuality and Reciprocity in Social Worker–Client Relationships: Rethinking Principles of Practice. *Journal of Social Work*, 9(1): 5–22.

Audre Lorde Quotes (nd) [online] Available at: www.brainyquote.com/citation/quotes/audre_lorde_390625 (accessed 28 September 2022).

Barsky, A (2018) Ethics Alive! Cultural Competence, Awareness, Sensitivity, Humility, and Responsiveness: What's the Difference? *The New Social*

Worker. [online] Available at: www.socialworker.com/feature-articles/eth ics-articles/ethics-alive-cultural-competence-awareness-sensitivity-humil ity-responsiveness/ (accessed 18 August 2022).

Bernhardt, B C and Singer, T (2012) The Neural Basis of Empathy. *Neuroscience*, 35(1): 1–23.

Bower, M and Solomon, R (eds) (2018) *What Social Workers Need to Know: A Psychoanalytic Approach*. Abingdon: Routledge.

British Association of Social Workers (BASW) (2021) The Code of Ethics for Social Work. [online] Available at www.basw.co.uk/about-basw/code-ethics (accessed 14 September 2022).

Dalai Lama (2018) *Human Values and Education*. Zurich: Zurich University of Applied Sciences.

Fewster, G (2004) Making Contact: Personal Boundaries in Professional Practice. *Related Child and Youth Care Practice*, 17(4): 8–18.

Fox et al (2014) Is Meditation Associated with Altered Brain Structure? A Systematic Review an Meta-analysis of Morphometric Neuroimaging in Meditation Practitioners. *Neuroscience & Biobehavioral Reviews* 43: 48–73.

Hardy, R (2018) Tips for Social Workers on Cultural Competence. *Community Care*. [online] Available at: www.communitycare.co.uk/2018/10/24/tips-social-workers-cultural-competence/ (accessed 18 August 2022).

Hingley-Jones, H and Ruch, G (2016) Stumbling Through? Relationship-Based Social Work Practice in Austere Times. *Journal of Social Work Practice*, 30(3): 235–48.

Howe, D (1998) Relationship-Based Thinking and Practice in Social Work. *Journal of Social Work Practice*, 12(1): 45–56.

Hozel, B K, Lazar, S W, Gord, T, Schuman-Olivier, Z, Vago, D R and Ott, U (2011) How Does Mindfulness Mediation Work? Proposing Mechanisms of Action from a Conceptual and Neural Perspective. *Perspectives on Psychological Science*, 6: 537–59.

Ingram, R and Smith, M (2018) Relationship-Based Practice: Emergent Themes in Social Work Literature. [online] Available at: www.iriss.org.uk/sites/default/files/2018-02/insights-41.pdf (accessed 20 September 2022).

Kabat-Zinn, J (nd) The Mindful Attitude of Trust. [online] Available at: https://mbsrtraining.com (accessed 18 August 2022).

Local Authority X v MM & Anor (2007) Court of Appeal, Family Division, 21 August.

Mayer, R C, David, J H and Schoorman, F D (1995) An Integrative Model of Organisational Trust. *Academy of Management Review*, 20: 709–34.

Nicholson, D and Artz, S (2003) Preventing Youthful Offending: Where Do We Go from Here? *Relational Child and Youth Care Practice*, 16(4): 32–46.

O'Leary, P, Tsui, M and Ruch, G (2013) The Boundaries of the Social Work Relationship Revisited: Towards a Connected, Inclusive and Dynamic Conceptualization. *British Journal of Social Work*, 43(1): 135–53.

Parker, S C, Nelson, B W, Epel, E S and Siegel, D J (2015) The Science of Presence: A Central Mediator of the Interpersonal Benefits of Mindfulness. In Brown, K W, Creswell, J D and Ryan, R M (eds) *Handbook of Mindfulness: Theory, Research & Practice* (pp 225–44). New York: Guildford Press.

Rousseau, D M, Sitkin, S B, Burt, R S, and Camerer, T (1998) Not So Different After All: A Cross-Discipline View of Trust. *Academy of Management Review*, 23(3): 393–404.

Ruch, G, Turney, D and Ward, A (2010) *Relationship-Based Social Work: Getting to the Heart of Practice*. London: Jessica Kingsley.

Shapiro, S L, Astin, J A, Bishop, S R and Cordova, M (2005) Mindfulness-based Stress Reduction for Health Care Professionals: Results from a Randomized Trial. *International Journal of Stress Management*, 12(2): 164–76.

Steadman, Y and Skaar, T (2019) Mindfulness, Trust and Leader Effectiveness: A Conceptual Framework. *Frontiers in Psychology*, 10: 1588. doi.org/10.3389/fpsyg.2019.01588

Tan, L B G, Yo, B C Y and Macrae, C N (2014) Brief Mindfulness Meditation Improves Mental State Attribution and Empathizing. *PLoS ONE*, 9(10): e110510.

Trevithick, P (2003) Effective Relationship-Based Practice: A Theoretical Exploration. *Journal of Social Work Practice*, 17(2): 163–76.

Ward, A (2018) The Use of Self. In Ruch, G, Turney, D and Ward, A (eds) *Relationship-Based Social Work: Getting to the Heart of Practice*. London: Jessica Kingsley.

Chapter 5

Assessment: the benefits of a mindful approach

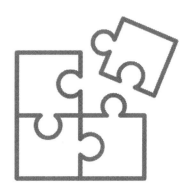

What one sees depends on where one looks

(Jones, 1983)

It seems that little can be done in social work without an assessment (McDonald, 2006). However, assessment is a nebulous term and concept, one that defies definition or standardisation. A rough definition of assessment in social work is that it is a method of collating information, analysing what has been gathered and using professional judgement to reach a decision about what kinds of intervention need to take place. This sounds like a simple process on paper, but in practice, managing the many composite parts can often become unwieldy, leading to outcomes that satisfy no one involved and which are often applied to a situation that has moved on significantly from where it was at the beginning of the assessment.

In this respect, assessment has always been an unsatisfactory tool in the social work inventory. Clearly, an evidence basis for provision of services or decisions that affect peoples' lives needs to be established, and the assessment model is a mechanism that can achieve this goal. If it is carried out well it can produce a record of how decisions were reached and note the input of all those who have an investment in a support or intervention taking place. It can become both an empowering process and document that provides an explicit rationale for the social worker/ service user relationship. However, when things go wrong, assessments are often found to be flawed, with difficulties arising from wrong or simply absent information, weak analysis or mistaken professional judgement. Helpful assessment formats and guidance have been introduced to mitigate the most prominent difficulties encountered by social workers. These serve to ensure a systematic, consistent approach to the appraisal of a person's life, but cannot replace the role of the social worker as self in the equation.

Good assessment also depends on the quality of the practice employed by the social worker (McDonald, 2006); formats, structures, knowledge and skills need to be deployed well by the practitioner in situ in order for them to create the most informative assessment, guiding successful action. This chapter reviews some of the pitfalls in this activity, seeking to highlight not where mindfulness replace social work guidance but where it can lend a hand to ease the process in the right direction.

This chapter will include:

Assessment framework

Bringing the person into view

Meeting the service user in the present

A key to unlocking partnership

Weighing the information

Analysis and judgement

Assessment framework

 Any social worker who has undertaken assessment work will recognise that it can become a juggernaut activity that consumes a large proportion of time. It can feel on occasion that social workers spend a disproportionate amount of their time assessing rather than intervening. Social workers are spread across a wide range of social work activities, including the assessment of risk, need, carers, mental capacity and for treatment or intervention, to name but a few. Notwithstanding their difference in functionality, assessments share a common purpose of helping someone to reach their potential by giving the right support at the right time to enable them to be safe, healthy and to live the life they choose.

Commonly, assessments need to include different aspects of a person's life. Often they are based on bio, psychosocial and possibly spiritual models, but ultimately they should extend beyond factual information and events to bring into focus the person themselves as the launch pad for any social work intervention that needs to take place. This brings into question what 'good' looks like within an activity in which very important, sometimes life changing decisions and action rest.

Historically, opinions are divided when it comes to the assessment approach. Many believe it to be a continuous process while at the same time recognising that it does not always present this way in practice (Payne, 2020). Others see assessment as a operating according to a very clear stage model (Milner and O'Bryne, 2020) illustrated below:

• preparation for the assessment

• collation of information

• critical reflection that involves the application of professional knowledge and analysis

• formation of professional judgement

• decision-making about recommendations and actions.

Both of these perspectives hold value, and it may be that the approach best adopted is one that fits the presenting situation as well as the professionals and service users involved. The idea of assessment as a continuous process will resonate with those who understand the ever-changing nature of people's circumstances, and this approach recognises that whatever approach is adopted, there needs to be awareness on the part of the social worker that there will have to be flexibility built into the activity. The approach that identifies explicit stages of the assessment process helps to tease out the components of a good assessment. Holding these elements in place mindfully helps to prevent procrastination or one's becoming adrift in a sea of information that is never effectually evaluated in order to lead to the next step in decision-making.

Bringing the person into view

 Mindful practice will enable the mindful social worker to keep sight of the assessment framework, allowing them to give consideration to the progress of each element while also noticing when the assessment might be moving away from its purpose or objective, at which point they can make adjustments to maintain its intended track. Application of mindful features can help to give shape to assessments in a way that brings the person being assessed into full view. This involves disruption of any tendency to apply habitual responses to information based on common experience, shifting instead to a more present awareness.

Mindful point of reflection

Before beginning an assessment of any kind, disrupt any tendency to lapse into a habitual, formulaic process; take some time to consider your approach in relation to the mindful fields in Figure 5.1.

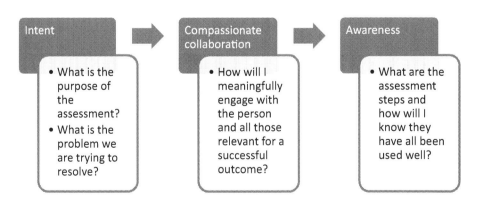

Figure 5.1 Adding a mindful perspective to assessment

Assessments need to include many different aspects of a person's life. In order to create a full picture for involvement, it can help to refer to life domains in order to make sure these are all taken into account (for example, individual, family, friends, wider support network, the community and culture). The ability of mindfulness to expand the view of the practitioner aids the mindful social worker in making sense of all of the available information. Restricting the opening of an assessment in order to focus on form-related enquiry provides only limited data about the person and their life, whereas starting with mindful curiosity in pursuit of a landscape view, as opposed to a narrow profile of a person's life, can lead to broader knowledge that can be discussed or clarified to provide the answers needed to establish a best course of action.

Practice example

Think of questions that might reflect a habitual response to assessment and those that might arise from mindful curiosity. Below are some examples. Which do you think might produce the landscape view?

- *So, Mr J, tell me what the problem is with your mobility.*

- *So, Mr J, tell me about yourself. How do you enjoy your day?*

- *Amy, tell me why you are unable to cope with your daughter Jo.*

- *Amy, can you describe to me how you find being a parent? Include what is good or challenging in order to help me understand your story.*

The landscape view arising from mindfulness provides greater insight into the situation being assessed, enabling more options for action to come into view. Secondly, it allows the social worker to show genuine interest in the other person, behaviour that will promote greater collaboration within an assessment, expanding the scope for action even further. And thirdly, it creates an assessment environment in which change can occur as a result of the assessment alone. As people talk more widely about themselves, they are also listening to their own narrative, and this can prompt realisations or insights about what needs to happen to bring into being the changes needed. This latter outcome also has the added benefit of empowering the service user to reach own solutions, building confidence, resilience and self-esteem along the way.

Assessment can be actively listening to what the client is asking, needing or wanting and meeting the client where they are with compassion and hope. It is the recognition of difference and being open to understand the other with a curiosity that invites a respectful exchange in order to provide best practice to those we serve.

(Clemons, 2014)

Meeting the service user in the present

One of the challenges of assessment is the constant change that is a feature of life; nothing stays the same for long, and this can result in assessment activity that takes place on shifting ground. While information about past behaviour acts as a guide to predict actions going forward, a mindful approach also holds in sight the present situation as it occurs. Mindful attention to the present enables decisions to be made based on the actuality of current events, creating a more solid foundation for assessments of risk or need, based on both historical and present awareness.

Practice example

Kate had grown up in the care system and was now a parent herself with two young daughters. Her daughters had become subject to a child-protection plan as Kate has had a series of short relationships with men who pose a risk to herself and her children. Kate has not always been attuned to the risks: her last partner of three months, Chris, was phys-ically violent to Kate and verbally aggressive to her daughters. Kate has now separated from this person. A child-protection review meeting was held to consider the children's removal from the child-protection plan into a position of voluntary support.

Professionals submitted their written reports the required 15 days before the meeting. All reports were positive, recognising the progress Kate had made in understanding the risks her partners had posed. The chair of the meeting began with an update from the social worker, who summarised her report. All professionals endorsed the situation with a view that the separation had been maintained and risk reduced. Kate was asked about the continued separation and she confirmed she had had no contact with Chris and would not engage if he tried to contact her.

→

A decision was made to remove the girls from the child-protection plan.

Just as everyone was leaving the meeting, Kate remarked to one of the school representatives that an old boyfriend of her youth had visited the previous evening, following a recent release from prison for offences of harassment of his former girlfriend. Kate believed him to be innocent of these offences and has allowed the friend to stay the night. She let him know that she would be happy to put him up for a few days.

In effect, the meeting had considered out-of-date information; decisions were being made entirely on past events without reference to the present. Consider what would have been different if the meeting had met the service user in the present, had started with an update from Kate rather than the social worker speaking from a report written 15 days earlier. The appraisal and decisions about risk would have been informed by meeting Kate in the present, enabling support to be tailored to current circumstances.

Life is not lived within a vacuum, it is a constant flow of activity. Mindful awareness of the ever-changing world allows the mindful social worker to understand the need to seek updates within a person's world, to check what has changed that might affect decisions or actions. Mindful attention to the present moment can help to avoid mistakes made on historic information alone, a preferable option to learning the lessons of hindsight when things have not turned out well due to an incomplete picture of events.

A key to unlocking partnership

 Assessments completed in isolation, without the genuine involvement of those who the social worker is trying to help, have diminished value in the wider scheme of decision-making. Working in partnership with those who use services is the ideal scenario, but barriers need to be overcome in order to achieve this goal in and of itself. Social workers must traverse a finely balanced course between closeness and distance, seeking alignment with the service user in order to be effective, but remaining sufficiently detached to prevent self-embroilment in the problem (Kettle, 2018). Sensitive management of the power differential is also required when seeking to unlock true partnership in assessment and intervention. Avoidance of the continual promotion of social work expertise in relation to the person or immersion in the person's difficulties, leading the social worker to resolve issues in the short term that do little to enhance the whole of the user's life for the better or to help them develop resilience for the future, requires mindful attention to how the social worker engages the person in the assessment. After all, this is the gateway activity to any further work, so how it is handled sets the tone for any future relationship or progress towards change.

Noticing the small as well as the big

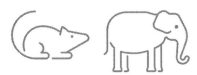 Working in a person-centred way is key to the formulation of assessment partnerships, and while assessments are directed at big questions about support, attention to detail, fostered by a mindful approach, is often the means of entry into valuable work to address what is at the heart of the social work engagement. The first encounter sets the precedent for things to come, putting the brakes on the bigger assessment agenda to give full attention to how at least the first encounter can go well. Attention to the small things can have the effect of creating a favourable environment for the rest of the task. *'Asking the client if there is anything else that might be helpful, is a collaborative effort acting on worth and dignity of all people, one of social work's central values'* (Kardushin, 1983). Mindful attention to these details of assessment in action can create change worthy of any content analysis. The mindful social worker retains awareness that assessment is intervention underway, and that acts of collaboration serve to help ease the process as well as build partnership and self-esteem and empower the service user.

Mindful point of reflection

Think of a time when a person did not make a good impression on you: What was the reason? Was it their manner, their presentation or because they were late and you felt they did not value your meeting?

It is these little things that can make the difference between an open or shut door into a person's life.

Bringing full awareness to the detailed planning of the nature of engagement with a person, as well as taking into account the work to be undertaken, can be a small thing that makes a big impact. Consider the examples below as illustrations of failure for want of mindful awareness of detail.

- Trying to talk to a mother about the safety of her children when the children have just arrived home from school hungry and in need of attention.

- Speaking to an older person in the lounge of a care home while background noise includes the radio, staff clattering trolleys for meals and a cleaner hovering nearby.

- Holding a meeting with a child service user in their school, because it is convenient for the professionals involved, when the site is the one place the child feels safe from their problems at home.

The actions above cannot hope to achieve a situation in which the service user is engaged on equal terms or where decision-making about how and when the work is carried out is shared on an equal basis. Shared engagement, fostered by attention to detail, is able to evoke change that can lead to parity in the assessment and collaboration that undoubtedly results in better outcomes.

While many valuable tools are available to aid person-centred practice, these can be under-utilised if there is a failure to engage with awareness in the present, with genuine curiosity about the person, their circumstances, hopes and dreams, or a lack of attention to opportunities to address risks and actions in a collaborative way. It is only by paying attention to how to genuinely engage with the service user that, as social workers, we can start the journey to understanding how best to work in a strengths-based, solution-focused partnership.

Practice example

Consider the two conversations below. The latter incorporates a mindful, present, curious approach. Which do you feel is the better conversation and why?

Paul has moved into a new supported-living accommodation. He is living with complex mental health problems. His support workers are concerned that he is not leaving his accommodation and seems to be becoming increasingly low in mood. He continually states that he misses his old flat and wants to go back there. This is not an option as the flat has been sold. Reith, Paul's social worker, visits Paul to find out how to help.

Conversation A

Reith has discussed the move with Paul and asks how he is feeling. Paul states he is low in mood and misses his old flat, but knows that returning is not an option. Reith asks Paul what his moods are like. Paul is non-communicative. Reith asks Paul if he would welcome a health appointment to discuss his medication. Paul responds that he will accept this. In the meantime, Reith suggests some social activities in the area that Paul might enjoy. Paul has the information and states he will think about it. There are also some mental health support groups that might help, and again Paul agrees to look at the information. Reith lets Paul know he will be back the following week.

Conversation B

Reith opens a conversation with Paul about how things are going. Paul states he is low in mood and misses his old flat, but knows that returning there is not an option. Reith acknowledges Paul's loss with empathy. Using genuine curiosity, Reith asks Paul what he liked about his old flat that he misses so much. Paul is uncertain at first, but Reith remains genuinely curious, prompting Paul for a description with mindful, intelligent, sensitive questioning. Paul describes the building, the space that he inhabited, his neighbours, the view and the area that he lived in. Reith persists in his curiosity, asking about details of each aspect, Paul particularly liked the park opposite his home. There is no park locally in the current accommodation. Curious pursuit of detail in the conversation helps Reith to identify that Paul enjoyed the flowers and shrubs in the park, most of which he could name. As the conversation progresses Reith notices the plants in the current flat and on the balcony.

Paul acknowledges the compliments that Reith gives to his current flat. As the conversation continues, Paul realises that he is missing green

$\longrightarrow$

space to enhance his mood. Reith and Paul are able to discuss how this aspect of his life could be accessed in his current accommodation. Both identify the communal green space in the current building and feel that there are possibilities for Paul to undertake some gardening work. Reith agrees to search out green-space opportunities locally, and Paul feels he is able to discuss use of the communal green space for growing things with the accommodation manager.

Reflect on the aspects of mindfulness that have aided this approach. How do the two versions of the conversation measure against success in the assessment of Paul's mental health needs?

An open, mindful approach, distinct from closed moments of habit that afflict us all, enables the mindful social worker to pursue conversational questions without already presuming the answers. It enables an assessment journey of authentic exploration of the circumstances, risks and strengths that reaches a real, shared commitment regarding the way forward, which differentiates this approach from any kind of superficial agreement about actions that the social worker thinks are best.

Weighing the information

 At some point, the information gathered during the assessment process will need to be analysed, with an ensuing judgement made about its meaning in relation to decisions and actions. If mindful awareness has been applied to the intent, the nature of the collaboration and the stages of work at the beginning of the assessment, it will be easier to determine when the analysis point naturally arises. However, attention to the shape of the assessment needs to be maintained lest the activity be lost in a continuous search or update of information to no end. Recognising the point at which analysis and judgement needs to occur is a particular skill that in itself involves a fine balance regarding the gathering of sufficient data on which to base a view, with events continuing and an ongoing need for outcomes. Mindful attention to both the form and the detail of the assessment, holding both in mind, will enable the mindful social worker to see the end point of information-gathering on the horizon, facilitating appropriate steps to bring the assessment to the analysis point.

Analysis and judgement

Analysis and judgement within assessment should be objective, fair and well balanced, drawing on the skills, experience and values of professional judgement, although the battle against the intrusion of personal or unconscious bias into professional judgement exists in the assessment arena, as it does all aspects of social work. Surfacing some of the pitfalls helps to bring them to out into the open so that they can be subjected to mindful reflection by the social worker in order to safeguard against undue personal bias influencing judgement at the point of assessment. *'When you begin paying attention to what's on your mind, you rapidly discover that everything is a judgment of one kind or another. It is good to be aware of this'* (Kabat-Zinn, 2006).

Revisiting culture

Approaching culture with humility, as discussed in Chapter 4, facilitates cultural competency within assessment. Accurate assessment requires that the assessor have an awareness of cultural difference and the part it plays in the path of successful assessment that is culturally appropriate in its application (Dean et al, 2006). Attunement to character traits derived from cultural context becomes vital to the correct identification of culturally appropriate intervention. Sensitivity to cultural reference facilitates greater insight into the presence of cultural bias in the assessment process, enabling recognition of incorrect assumptions that can be harmful to the person receiving services. The mindful social worker is able to hold this awareness in mind while carrying out assessment activities, baking in cultural self-reflection in moments of pause during information-gathering and analysis.

A mindful, culturally alert social worker will have in view their own cultural values and biases and knowledge of their service users' worldviews, and will possess intervention strategies and culturally alert skills (McAuliffe et al, 2008; Clemens, 2014).

But mindful meditation extends this quality to the non-judgemental aspects of character that help the practitioner to resist leaps to unconscious bias in their work. Research by Lueke and Gibson (2014) supports a link between mindfulness and a reduction in bias in relation to both age and race. A group of participants who took part in the study received ten-minute mindfulness exercises, and subsequently showed less bias regarding race and age in implicit-association tests than those in the control group, who didn't received mindfulness practice. Participants were asked to align positive or negative words with black or white faces and old or young faces. Those who had completed mindfulness exercises showed less automatic activation of negative associations (for example, that black is bad, or that old is bad) than those in the control group. Even more remarkable was the fact that the mindful participants exhibited this reduction in bias without even focusing on the biases themselves, and also showed less delineation of the faces into categories of black, white, old or young, resisting the habit of expectation response. *'The ability to curb implicit bias and weaken negative association by being more mindful could help prevent all kinds of negative effects'* (Torres, 2014).

The ability to reduce automatic responses enables greater objectivity to be present, making room for observation of the unique situation before us rather than reliance on established patterns of association that can rest on unsound foundations. This increases the quality of attention in the assessment procedure, making sure that the whole picture is observed and assessed with no presumptuous shortcuts taken.

Further bumps in the road

 There are a number of other pitfalls to look out for when conducting an assessment, and while it may not always be possible to avoid or eliminate them, mindful attention to some of the things that can unduly influence assessment, particularly analysis and judgement, can be a first step towards a balanced, fair and accurate outcome.

Kirkman and Melrose (2014) identified many of the common challenges to achieving balance in assessments through their research into clinical judgement and decision-making in children's social work. Many will be familiar to social work professionals, particularly if any attention has been given to serious case review.

• Example bias: social workers can make judgements about the prob-ability of events based on how easy it is to bring examples of the event occurring to mind. For example, older people frequently fall and incur injury, ergo it is considered probable that an older person will fall. Or a mother under stress smacks a child, therefore it is considered likely that if a parent is under stress they will smack their child.

- Confirmation bias: only looking for evidence that confirms pre-existing views. A social worker views an adult with a disability as unable to cope, and therefore fails to see the strengths the adult displays in managing their life.

- Groupthink: the occurrence of bias when there is collective problem-solving and a desire to avoid conflict and achieve unanimity becomes a significant driver that can result in bad decision-making. For example, a looked after review decision that siblings should be separated because one exhibits challenging behaviour that might impact the stability of the placement for both.

- Relative judgement: social workers judge cases in comparison to others because it is cognitively easier to do so. For example, the expectation that an older person living at home with dementia will inevitably need residential care as this is what has happened in similar cases.

- Decision avoidance: instances when the emotional nature of an event leads to delaying or avoidance of the most appropriate decision (for example, the removal of a child from a family home).

- Reference reluctance: a reluctance to question the authority of a source of information can lead to ill-judged weight being assigned to the report. For example, the reluctance to challenge authority highlighted in the serious case review of Victoria Climbié demonstrated the importance of challenging established medical views.

- Tunnel vision: adopting the first suitable course of action rather than taking opportunities to compare and consider options.

Practice example

Consider two accounts of a father's relationship with his daughter. Which of the pitfalls do you think the social worker might have fallen into? How might mindful reflection help to correct the balance?

A social worker records that a father is always late for contact with his child. She feels this is an indication that he is not committed to seeing his daughter. He often leaves early and sometimes does not attend at all,

→

failing to let the social worker know. She has concluded that the father does not wish to take care of his child, that his lifestyle is erratic, as he cannot adhere to simple contact times, and that he is hostile to working with professionals as he does not communicate when he is not attending. Her experience is that this is not an unusual state of affairs in relation to children in care.

A foster carer views a father as very engaged with his daughter: he always phones at the time and day agreed, and she can tell that his daughter enjoys the conversations and always feels happy afterwards. The foster carer is aware that the father is looking for work so that he can rent a flat to create a home for his daughter, but his employment search sometimes means he has been unable to attend face-to-face contact with his daughter at the social services offices. When he does attend, he has to leave early sometimes to catch a bus, and the foster carer thinks it might be helpful if she could give him a lift or if social services could arrange transport. The foster carer understands this, as she herself has problems contacting the social worker or getting messages through. The father has also let her know that he has had difficulty contacting the social worker to let her know he will not be attending at short notice, and he does not think the messages are being passed on.

Mindfulness enables the mindful social worker to counteract and disrupt these unhelpful tendencies that pervade assessment and decision-making. It teaches the practitioner to approach each event with a new mind, one that can help to discard the example and confirmation bias that can so easily cloud judgement. It promotes pause and self-reflection during assessment in order to recognise and counterbalance any instances when unconscious bias might be taking place, prompting intelligent review of self in action and noticing the values, attitudes and beliefs that are coming into play in the analysis of information and the basis of decision-making. The mindful skill of self-regulation, reducing unhelpful emotive responses to emotionally challenging situations and ensuring any conclusions or actions are not hindered by an emotive response that does not always lead to right course of action. also mitigates the challenge of decision avoidance highlighted by Kirkman and Melrose (2014). Mindful awareness combats the tendency towards tunnel vision, ensuring an expansive approach is applied to assessment, one that includes a broader understanding as well as the details of particular issues. It is this more expansive lens that can encourage the mindful social worker to incorporate the wider social justice dynamic into an assessment (for example, how human rights or social injustices such as poverty, poor education or poor healthcare impact the nature and type of intervention needed).

Practice example

Consider once more the case scenario provided in the previous practice example, the two perspectives on a father's engagement in contact arrangements for his daughter and his commitment to her return to his care. A broader awareness will not only include the actions of the father in response to the contact arrangements but will also consider the issues the father is dealing with in terms of employment, suitable accommodation and travel arrangements. The social work intervention will not only include terms of contact but also how to redress some of the social problems the father is facing in order to achieve the outcome of reunification between father and daughter, an outcome both parties want and need for their well-being.

Take-home message

Good assessment and decision-making must include not only attention to the external information and reflection but also mindful attention to self in action as part of the assessment dynamic.

Assessments are complex activities that incorporate so much that is explicit and implicit about information, emotions, behaviours and purpose. Giving the process one's full attention can be difficult, and guarding against bias or unhelpful influences that render assessments unfair or unjust can be even harder. The consequences of the resulting analysis and decision-making can be life-changing, so doing all to enable a good assessment is crucial. Mindfulness lends itself as an obvious tool to support the mindful social worker in this pivotal action, both by shifting to a broad lens through which to encompass the whole picture and in helping to instill reflection and time for pause in the activity in order to increase accuracy, insight and balance. Mindfulness could be the tool that puts the breaks on the out-of-control train of assessment in order to steer it onto the right track to achieve the outcomes needed.

Takeaways

1. Key points

- Assessment is a core social work activity that needs full attention.

- The varied nature and purpose of assessment means it is an activity that defies a universal format, relying instead on the knowledge, skill and judgement of the social worker performing the task.

- Assessment is a continuous activity that needs to be responsive to the ever-changing world, an approach encouraged by mindful practice.

- Assessment needs the assessor to discard tunnel vision and automatic thinking to broaden their awareness; mindfulness promotes this broader perspective.

- A mindful approach to establishing an authentic partnership within assessment can be transformational for reaching assessment goals, those that are both expected and unexpected but valued nonetheless.

- Assessment can constitute truly, professionally objective non-judgemental collation, analysis and action only through the noticing of self in action. Mindfulness nurtures this self-observation, protecting against the presence of unconscious bias.

- Mindfulness creates a pause that shifts practice away from habitual reactivity, whereby assessment merely confirms a prejudged outcome, towards a true reflection of the service user's life, needs, risks, strengths and goals.

2. Mindful self in action: Assessments reflection tool

'I consider each assessment as a unique, without pre-judgement about the outcome.'

'I use research and evidence to inform assessment outcomes.'

'I listen without judgement or bias.'

'I check the foundation of any thinking to avoid groupthink. I ask questions about things I do not understand.'

'I plan assessments with attention to the authentic involvement of the persons involved.'

'I take mindful pauses to check my own attitudes and behaviours relative to the assessment content and direction.'

'I mindfully return to self during assessment activity to maintain social work values, honesty, accountability and partnership.'

3. Culturegram

Culturegrams were created by Dr Elaine Congress, a member of the International Federation of Social Work, who felt that ecomaps and genograms did not go far enough to help us understand culture, particularly for those who migrate and are new to their countries of residence.

The following fields constitute the essential elements of information for understanding a given service user's culture:

- reason for relocation;

- legal status;

- time in the community;

- language spoken at home and in the community;

- health beliefs;

- impact of trauma and crisis events;

- contact with cultural and religious institutions, holidays, food and clothing;

- experiences of discrimination, oppression, bias and racism;

- values about education and work;

- values about family structure, power, myths and rules.

References and further reading

Bonnick, H (2006) Frontlines: Developing Non-Judgmental Issues. *Community Care*. [online] Available at: www.communitycare.co.uk/2006/05/11/frontlines-developing-non-judgemental-issues/ (accessed 18 August 2022).

Clemons, J (2014) *Client System Assessment Tools for Social Work Practice*. North American Association of Christians in Social Work. [online] Available at: www.academia.edu/29776169/CLIENT_SYSTEM_ASSESSMENT_TOOLS_FOR_SOCIAL_WORK_PRACTICE (accessed 6 September 2022).

Dean, H, Hepworth, R, Rooney, R, Dewberry, G, Rooney, K, Gottfried, S and Larson, J (2006) *Direct Social Work Practice: Theory and Skills*. Belmont, CA. Thomson Brooks.

Jones, C (1983) *State Social Work and the Working Class*. London: Macmillan.

Kabat-Zinn, J (2006) *Mindfulness for Beginners*. Colorado: Sounds True Publications.

Kadushin, A (1983) *The Social Work Interview*. New York: Columbia University Press.

Kirkman, E and Melrose, K (2014) *Clinical Judgement and Decision Making in Children's Social Work: An Analysis of the 'Front Door' System*. [online] Available at: https://assets.publishing.service.gov.uk/government/uploads/system/uploads/attachment_data/file/305516/RR337_-_Clinical_Judgement_and_Decision-Making_in_Childrens_Social_Work.pdf (accessed 18 August 2022).

Lueke, A and Gibson, B (2014) Mindfulness Meditation Reduces Implicit Age and Race Bias. *Social Psychological and Personality Science*, 6(3): 284–91.

McAuliffe, G (ed) (2008) *Culturally Alert Counseling: A Comprehensive Introduction*. Thousand Oaks, CA: Sage.

Milner, J and O'Bryne, P (2020) *Assessment in Social Work*, 5th edition. Basingstoke: Palgrave Macmillan.

Payne, M (2020) *Modern Social Work Theory*, 5th edition. London: Bloomsbury Academic.

Richmond, M E (1917) *Social Diagnosis.* New York: Russell Sage Foundation.

Torres, N (2014) Mindfulness Mitigates Bias You May Not Know You Have. *Harvard Business Review*. [online] Available at: https://hbr.org/2014/12/mindfulness-mitigates-biases-you-may-not-know-you-have#:~:text=Research%20on%20overcoming%20implicit%20age%20and%20racial%20bias.&text=Researchers%20can't%20seem%20to,working%20memory%2C%20and%20increased%20compassion (accessed 18 August 2022).

Chapter 6

Mindfulness, creativity and problem-solving

We have more possibilities in each moment that we realise.

(Nhat Hanh, 2007)

It is no accident that Silicon Valley has embraced mindfulness as a priority on their list of corporate activities. Google promote an internal mindfulness programme that encourages workers to complete mindful activities to enhance their performance at work (Parlerisa, 2019), while Twitter and Facebook have also introduced contemplative practice, *'holding regular in office meditation "sessions" and arranging work routines to maximise mindfulness'* (Shachtan, 2013). It seems that many companies, including those in the tech industry, are recognising the contribution mindfulness can make to creative ideas and new ways of thinking that support the effectiveness of the business world.

Social work, by its very nature, demands similar levels of creativity, requiring social workers to *'contribute to an open and creative learning culture in the workplace to discuss, reflect on and share best practice'* (Social Work England, 2022). Its focus on people as individuals, balancing the need for support alongside recognition and management of risk, requires innovative thought with creative solutions to produce positive transformation.

While not seeking to replace the requirement for evidence-based practice using established interventions, Silicon Valley demonstrates that mindfulness can bring something extra to the worktable. This is as true for social work as it is anywhere else. The achieving of mind hygiene through mindfulness practice can promote greater flexibility of thought, increased divergent thinking and greater aptitude for problem-solving (Colzato et al, 2012; Ostafin and Kashan, 2012). Put simply, *'learning to enhance and increase engagement and be in the moment with clients increases your ability to innovate'* (Jackson, 2020).

This chapter will include:

What do we mean by creativity and what does it look like?

Opportunities for creativity in the social work role

Building creative credentials through mindfulness

Insight problem-solving

Applying mindfulness to problem-solving

Social work is often described as one of the helpful or caring professions, but these limited labels belie the breadth of what social work can do, the nature of the role and the demands that it makes, all of which require, in varying degrees, creativity, a characteristic that should definitely be included in the adjective mix when describing the nature of the profession. This chapter looks at the shape of creativity within social work and the impetus to develop our professional and personal creativity to meet the challenges of the role.

What do we mean by creativity and what does it look like?

I've looked it up, so you don't have to

 Traditionally, our touchstone when referencing creativity might be the arts, bringing to mind those talented individuals who produce beautiful works of art, living performances of drama or street work, taking creative, artistic expression to levels that lead to wonder and admiration from those who have not developed this ability or talent. But creativity lives within everyone and can be expressed in many different ways of living, including in the workplace. Its recognition and use is also really good for well-being, producing feelings of relaxation, satisfaction and happiness alongside its benefits for those around us.

With regard to creativity in the workplace, the following description might help us understand its relevance.

> Creativity is defined as the tendency to generate or recognise ideas, alternatives or possibilities that may be useful in solving problems and communication with others.
>
> To be creative you need to be able to view things in new ways or from a different perspective you need to be able to generate new possibilities or new alternatives.

(Franken, 2006, p 334)

Franken goes on to make the point that creative ability is linked to other traits, such as flexibility, tolerance of ambiguity or unpredictability, all of which are very much needed to sustain the social work role.

The gift that keeps on giving

 It seems that as we use and develop our creativity, things just get better. Richard N Foster (2015) points out that the creative process is iterative rather than linear, that when we have one new idea, it often inspires others in a connected way. Creativity is a win-win activity that produces happiness and well-being for ourselves as well as for those around us, including our work colleagues and those whom we seek to support.

Take-home message

Creativity generates new perspectives, ideas and possibilities. It is innate within us all, and the more we use it, the better it gets for everyone.

Opportunities for creativity in the social work role

Whether you have been practising for a while or have just become a social worker, opportunities for creativity soon become apparent as you juggle different perspectives and bespoke interventions that are needed to meet the variety of circumstances encountered. Reflection on the issue of creativity shines a light on just how much there is a need for creativity in the social work role, raising the query as to why it is not given more attention within professional development; there is a long way to go to catch up with Silicon Valley.

Social work is not a one-size-fits-all activity; while we may encounter similar problems often in similar contexts, the requirement to work with individuals or families as they present themselves demands that social workers draw from a range of responses that need, by the nature of interactions, to be flexible and adaptive, indeed creative. Personalised, effective management of self as an essential social work resource requires creative skill in order to meet the unique, complex life situations that arise within practice. Good communication that leads to the building of trusted relationships, often originating from a poor starting point given people's vulnerabilities, demands a creative approach. Imagination needs to be in play to be able to view the world from different perspectives, most importantly from the perspective of those we seek to support. Creative thinking also helps to crystallise information gathered into plans that will work in the complex human world.

When met with hostility or refusal to engage, the ability to reflect on creative ways to open the door to partnership allows the social worker to make progress where otherwise there might be roadblocks. The opportunities for creative thinking are numerous and a lengthy review of the social work role will probably lead to our identifying many more aspects that rely on a creative nature, including yet more areas where social workers encourage service users' creativity to help build on strengths to support well-being. 'Social work in fact demands the... constant need for creative response to poorly understood problems' (Clark, 1995).

The constant dynamic between social and medical models of practice, in the context of the recent historic tendency to add process and bureaucracy to social work, may have had the effect of throwing the creative baby out with the bathwater. By seeking to impose consistency and avoid mistakes that are often costly in terms of human impact, social work has (to a degree) lost the element of creativity that facilitates flexibility in tailored responses to individual models of living.

Throughout history, there has been an ongoing tension between the various domains of social work activity, most prevalently between science and art, and in particular regarding the application of either a social or medical model and the difficulties in balancing prescriptive ways of working (aiming to help the social worker avoid mistakes) alongside a social-composite model that is more closely aligned with a person-centred approach. Indeed, the emphasis on procedure at the expense of creativity can only further restrict personalised practice, perhaps by limiting managed risk, but also by stifling the wider role of the social worker as an arbiter of social change, a champion of rights in the face of social injustice. However, change is afoot with the adoption of a different approach in recent years. Increasingly, working methodologies and conversations are focusing on the benefits of the creative aspects of the social work role, finding a way to redress the balance between compliance and creativity, the latter being essential to supporting the strengths-based, solution-focused approaches of the current social work era. *'Social workers need the space to be creative, to make use of their experience and to act according to case-by-case judgments'* (McFarlane, 2017).

McFarlane goes on to provide an example of a local authority, Hackney Council, reviewing their paperwork and processes to enable greater space for social workers to engage their creativity. This is credited with halving social workers' sickness absence and reducing the population of looked-after children by at least 40 per cent; food for thought within a profession that has high levels of stress and limited resources due to service user need.

Take-home message

Creativity is an integral part of social work, just as much as in other professions; tapping into our creativity credentials might be just the thing needed to boost intervention in the right direction for those who use services.

Building creativity credentials through mindfulness

While creativity has become the much sought-after holy grail of many businesses and public services, little attention is paid to how creativity can in fact be encouraged, developed or nurtured in the working environment. It is commonly agreed that creativity is innate within us all; it is a natural feature of humanity, designed to assist adaptation to the inevitably changing world, to aid survival in the face of adversity by helping us overcome problems with what often become pretty clever solutions.

The burgeoning power of creativity can be witnessed in our living world, particularly in response to crisis situations such as the Covid-19 pandemic or climate change.

But there remains a difficulty as to how organisations can support creative expansion: often there is a drive to employ new people, possibly leaning towards the young, who are deemed to have not yet formed solid, habitual thought patterns about specific work roles, or to drive creativity through the employment of those who have already demonstrated their creative credentials. Unfortunately, unless there is a cultural drive towards creativity, often these champions merely become absorbed into the prescriptive approaches of their organisations, with creative thinking sacrificed to process.

However, mindfulness can offer a bridge to the initiation and recovery of creative thinking, in support of both personal and professional adaptability and flexibility. The value of mindfulness is being realised not only in relation to well-being but in terms of its contribution to our creative powers. The practice itself centres around the reduction of internal, verbal dialogue that encourages stress, anxiety and depressive thoughts. As this internal state becomes quiet, space is made available for creativity, fostering traits that support the creative process.

Mindfulness and creativity as natural bedfellows

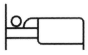

Mindfulness not only engenders in its practitioners a stronger resistance to established patterns or familiar rules in routine situations, it also provides the mindful social worker with the ability to transcend the need to reassuringly join up the dots of experience in an established way. Mindful awareness enables one to break free from habitual ways of thinking and enables novelty to emerge (Moore and Malinowski, 2009).

The positive effects of mindful meditation encompass both divergent and convergent thinking to support creativity. Research by Colzato et al (2012) highlights the presence of enhanced divergent thinking through mindfulness, indicative of the raising of numerous pathways of solutions for problem-solving. This way of thinking is particularly helpful for social work due to its facilitating the creative growth of options and opportunities that offer the service user choice and control over the next steps in problem-solving. As such, mindful practice has the potential to support a movement of social work away from the frustrating one-size-fits-all, resource-led approach and towards a more creative, strengths-based practice that focuses on bespoke connections and solutions that can be determined by individuality. Mindful meditation has also been observed to enhance positive mood, a further lever for divergent thinking and subsequent inventive creativity.

Mindfulness generates a more measured approach to social work, ensuring there is less quick judgement or reactive evaluation, allowing a gap to emerge, one that allows for greater insight, supporting more innovative conversation while also increasing practitioners' attentiveness to the ordinary in a way that might lead to creativity in problem-resolution. Carson and Langer (2006) draw attention to the capacity of mindfulness to open the mind to new possibilities, to alter perspectives, and in doing so to expand the range of possible responses to many of social work's most difficult situations.

Mindful point of reflection

Think of a time when you had problem-solving moment or idea; this is your creativity gene activating. What made it happen? How did it help you or others? How did it make you feel? By mindfully noticing these events, we can help them to reoccur, enhancing our ability to develop new ideas and ways of thinking.

Insight problem-solving

The relationship between mindfulness and creativity also enhances the skill of insight problem-solving. This creative ability is of obvious use within social work, a profession that seeks to resolve difficulties while also ensuring good outcomes for people involved with services.

What is insight problem-solving?

Insight problem-solving is often described as that 'Aha!' or 'Eureka!' moment of reaching a solution. Non-insight problem-solving can be said to involve a linear set of defined steps that should logically lead to resolution and which have been proven over time as established, accepted learning. Insightful solutions to problem responses are required when the usual responses do not apply or do not reach a satisfactory resolution. It is at these times that we become blocked and reach a point of stagnation, leading to confusion and frustration. This can further lead to despondency, a sense of failure, withdrawal from solution-seeking and one's tolerating the problem even as it may become worse. This situation must be familiar to many social workers, who are faced with complex difficulties that seem to defy logical understanding, sometimes generating anxiety or fear about the risks to an individual as the problems escalate. This frustration and perceived blockage may be the result of overreliance on habitual solutions or intense focus on inappropriate cues (Sandkühler and Bhattacharya, 2008). It is often something that is noticed with hindsight or as the result of serious case review when a person has died or been seriously injured and more could have been done by professionals to prevent such an event.

Thinking outside the box or even with no box at all

 Insight problem-solving begins with taking a much broader approach to the problem, entertaining more than one perspective or method of solution. Often the point of most frustration when seeking a solution is the point at which our minds trigger the need to consider different approaches; it is then that the problem is looked at with fresh eyes, leading to a subconscious experience of a creative solution where none could previously be seen. This unconscious process involves a reshuffling of information or factors deep within the subconscious mind, which enables us to make connections that our conscious, logical, habitual mind inhibited us from making (Schooler et al, 1993). In fact, triggering our insight-problem-solving creativity enables us to think outside the box, or to go one step further and think with no box present at all.

A famous example of insight problem-solving

In 1854, an outbreak of cholera occurred in Broad Street, London, killing more than 600 people. The outbreak was part of a worldwide spread of the disease and was not uncommon. The established, habitual thinking of the time was that the disease was spread by 'miasma', foul-smelling air result from rotting material in the streets.

However, insight problem-solving utilised by Dr John Snow found a different story. He concluded that the disease was transmitted by water-borne bacteria: germs. His observation of the use of a water pump in the area enabled him to support his new hypothesis, identifying the pump as the source of infection and resulting in a reduction in infection when the water pump handle was removed. A simple solution to a deadly disease.

The insight problem-solving of Dr Snow led to fundamental changes in the water and waste systems of London as well as around the country, and significant public-health improvements both nationally and internationally, knowledge that continues to apply to the present world.

The value of insight problem-solving for social work

Many case reviews when someone has died or been seriously injured highlight failings as a result of habitual thinking: process-driven actions that lead a social worker to fail to notice or perceive what is actually happening while they are helping a service user. Insight problem-solving enables social workers to see situations from different perspectives, providing the opportunity to make unique connections. Such a creative process can, when one is working closely with adults, families and children alongside partner agencies, result in genuine, solution-focused approaches. This enacts the very aim of most social work direction, that of treating the individual and circumstances afresh without attempting to impose a one-size-fits-all solution on the issues as they arise. The use of a mindful approach that encourages insight means that social workers are responsive to bureaucratic process but not trapped by it. The application of mindfulness to this area leads to intelligent evaluation rather than quick judgements, careful, insightful planning rather than reactive knee-jerk responses, and concentration not only on what needs to be done but on the *way* it needs to be done in collaboration in order to foster empowerment for the future.

Practice example

The concept of harm through coercion is a relatively recent example of insight problem-solving, originating out of observation and from a review of instances when people have been injured by coercive activity, whether by a relative or close friend or a stranger. Professionals developed insight into the issue by entertaining different possibilities about why a person may not accept support or make choices that place them at risk. Insight problem-solving emerged in the techniques used to engage the victims not only in actions to improve safety but also to manage relationships where the coercer was a significant person in the victim's life and where ongoing relations might need to continue.

Mindfulness insight supports the social work approach of treating people with humanity, recognising their multifaceted personhood and allowing the social worker to see the whole picture rather than a particular problematic aspect of it. As such, it is a piece of the supporting architecture for strengths-based, solution-focused work that asks us to consider all that is important or of value to the service user within the context in which they live. In turn, this recognition opens up a greater number of possibilities for the way positive life changes might be achieved. Deeper conversations can take place that focus not only on immediate safety and well-being but extend to the user's aspirations for the future, devising how decisions can be taken that create conditions for such aspirations to come to fruition. A levelling-up occurs in the power relationship between social worker and service user, which in turn supports increased collaboration that gives rise to creative thinking about the best way to achieve a good life. Again, this engenders choice and greater equality of power between social worker and service user, as a route towards positive change is agreed and navigated.

Practice example

A strong example of insight problem-solving within the social justice context is exhibited in the University of Chichester's project to support people who are homeless to access university education. Becky Edwards, an employee of the university, developed a course module to support people who are homeless to develop the confidence and skills to apply for a degree course. Edwards was struck by the difference between being intelligent and being educated. This indeed seems to have been her insight 'Aha!' moment. She believed many who were homeless or vulnerable were intelligent but suffered from the absence of education. Edwards' insight problem-solving took the form of establishing the hypothesis that just because these people were not educated did not mean they were not capable of achieving academic success. Her creative insight went further when she designed the module with the input of homeless people to ensure that it met individual needs.

We are using lived experience to develop academic reading, writing and research skills, self-confidence, self-esteem and self-belief. Honest and insightful links are made between themes like emotional intelligence, reflective practice, decision making skills critical thinking and past often painful experiences.

(Edwards, 2019)

The university-access example encapsulates all that might be possible through insight creativity. Mindfulness can nurture this aspect of our person to empower social workers to make increased use of their creative character, aiming practice at an inspiring community level as well as meeting individual needs. Mindfulness insight enables social workers to look at the issues affecting those accessing services with a broader lens, including and extending beyond case work to the wider context of social injustice and inequality. This guides social workers to more fruitfully engage not only with casework but also with the advocacy of social justice, an important element of the role often subservient to the presenting issues of each case as they consume attention. It places the social work gaze within the wider picture, where social workers can encourage disadvantaged groups to advocate for themselves to resolve wider community problems while also acting as champions on their behalf.

Applying mindfulness to problem-solving

Research suggests that building a base layer of mindful practice in your life enhances creative problem-solving abilities. This base layer need only consist of short periods of meditation or quiet mind-clearing, practised regularly to develop increased skill in this area. Mindfulness gives rise to self-regulation, and this becomes relevant to problem-solving in social work when situations of intransigence or stagnation in practice arise. Often this is the cause of frustration that others, such as professionals or service users, do not view the situation or solutions from the same perspective as we do. Accusations of manipulation or unacceptable risk-taking can arise from our own anxieties or fears for the people involved or of concerns about our own actions.

A mindful approach encourages self-monitoring in such encounters, noticing the frustrations that occur but taking moments to understand the cause and effect of such feelings. A mindful social worker is able to take a step back to consider the situation anew, examining not only external events but also the role of self, both professional and personal, in relation to the lack of progress in a case. This ability to detach, to look afresh at perspectives, weigh different narratives for the difficulties encountered, triggers the creative self to address the issues in a different way, to move around or over the roadblock rather than continue to try to move it with force. *'Specifically experienced meditators are better problem solvers and have better verbal creativity'* (Henrikson et al, 2020).

Practice example

Take some quiet time to clear your mind and think creatively about how to engage Jack.

Jack is 50 years old and reports that he does sometimes have mental health issues, which manifest as periods of manic activity followed by depression. He is happy to take some medication, but often does not like how it makes him feel and will sometimes stop. Jack enjoys collecting things, and this has resulted in boxes of items obstructing his bathroom, lounge and kitchen facilities. Neighbours have reported vermin within the area and believe that they are caused by a pile of rubbish building in Jack's garden. Jack has some mobility problems, and the boxes do restrict his movement, but he states that he is perfectly happy and does not need any help. The fire service

→

> *have raised concerns about fire risk, particularly in relation to Jack's ability to leave the home in an emergency. Jack is adamant he does not want to engage with any services and will not respond to social work visits.*

Rather than responding habitually, mindfulness can help us notice the basis for our response, in this case allowing us not only to see the difficulties in Jack's situation but also to understanding what needs to be in place in order for self as resource to intervene. A mindful social worker recognises what knowledge and support is required across the professional spectrum to engage successfully with the service user, and is able to provide meaningful supervision that will induce reflection about how best to act, alongside managing emotions regarding safety and risk. Rather than engaging in a continued battle with the service user about engagement, this mindful approach can encourage distance from the problem in order to think about the situation anew allowing space for creative solutions to arise, for fractious professional and service user relationships to be repaired and for the work to forge ahead on a more positive pathway.

A mindful approach allows us to hold different explanations for a situation in mind, and this is important when working to achieve well-being or resolve risk.

Mindful creativity, harnessed within the social work professional framework, has much to recommend it. Mindful enhancement of our innate creative abilities can be the impetus needed to enable our social work practice to 'catch fire' in regard to how we collaborate in order to attain bespoke solutions that really do meet the needs of those we work with both individually and in the wider social justice arena.

Takeaways

1. Key points

- The creativity gene exists within us all, and mindfulness can help us to switch it on.

- Creativity is not only for artists, it has relevance for social work in the way we engage, act and solve problems.

- Creativity used well serves both our well-being and the well-being of others.

- The more we flex our creative muscle, the more new ideas, perspectives and solutions we find.

- Mindfulness can unlock our creative nature, allowing it to grow in all that we do. It can lead to increased flexibility and adaptability and make us more agile or responsive in our social work practice.

- Mindfulness supports our capacity for insight problem-solving, enabling us to refresh our understanding of problems when we are stuck. This can be the key to unlocking the way forward, perhaps in a different direction.

- The mindful social worker who models creativity and insight problem-solving can commute these talents to service users, empowering them to experience the benefits of using creativity to resolve issues, with the added benefit of building confidence, self-esteem and resilience for the future.

2. Switching on the creative, insight problem gene

A good, mindful way of switching on the creative aspect of self, especially when immersed in an intransigent situation or problem, is to use the STOP approach as follows:

Table 6.1

Stop	Stop what you are doing.
Take a breath	Go for a walk, make a cup of tea or get some rest.
Observe	Notice your thoughts or feelings about the event. Observe if there is anything else you need to know, any useful questions you could ask, checks you could make. Are there any other ways of looking at the situation?
Proceed	Decide on a course of action. Give yourself plenty of options or alternatives. Take time to weigh the advantages or disadvantages of what you are doing. Know that you are moving forward with a non-reactive, balanced approach.

3. Cultivate humility to allow creativity to occur

Over-confidence, arrogance and a *'That's the way we do things around here'* approach are all factors that inhibit the growth of creativity. To notice new ideas or develop new ways of thinking, each situation has to be encountered as new, providing much to learn from, otherwise our over-confidence or established ways of doing things limit our view of all that might be possible. Clinging to patterns of work or a set way of carrying out tasks does not prevent change but does prevent flexibility to deal with change. Take time during a mindfulness or meditation session to notice humility; notice what thoughts occur, if your angry thoughts are about people not recognising your expertise or point of view. Focus on the feelings that arise and then allow them to disperse, accepting your own lack of knowledge and that there are many different ways of seeing things, all of which can provide creative learning.

References and further reading

Brown, K W, Ryan, R M and Cresswell, J D M (2007) Mindfulness: Theoretical Foundations and Evidence for Its Salutary Effects. *Psychological Inquiry*, 18(4): 211–37.

Carson, S and Langar, E (2006) Mindfulness and Self-Acceptance. *Journal of Rational Emotive and Cognitive Behaviour Therapy*, 24(1): 29–43.

Clark, C (1995) Competence and Discipline in Professional Formation. *British Journal of Social Work*, 25(5): 563–80.

Colzato, L S, Ozturk, A and Hommel, B (2012) Meditate to Create: The Impact on Focused-Attention and Open-Monitoring Training on Convergent and Divergent Thinking. *Frontiers in Psychology*, 3: 116.

Edwards, B (2019) University Can Change Homeless Peoples' Lives, but They Need Support to Get There. *The Guardian*, 18 April.

Foster, R N (2015) What Is Creativity? *Yale Insights*. [online] Available at: https://insights.som.yale.edu/insights/what-is-creativity (accessed 18 August 2022).

Franken, R E (2006) *Human Motivation*, 3rd edition. Belmont, CA: Thomson Wadsworth.

Henriksen, D, Richardson, C and Shack, K (2020) Mindfulness and Creativity: Implications for Thinking and Learning. *Thinking Skills and Creativity*, 37: 100689. doi:10.1016/j.tsc.2020.100689

Jackson, K (2020) The Mindful Social Worker: How Mindfulness Can Help Social Workers Practice More Creatively. *Social Work Today*, 17(5): 14.

McFarlane, D (2017) We Need to Engage and Motivate Social Workers – Lets Get Creative. *The Guardian*, 25 January.

Moore, A and Malinowski, P (2009) Meditation, Mindfulness and Cognitive Flexibility. *Consciousness and Cognition*, 18(1): 176–86.

Nhat Hanh, T (2007) *The Art of Power*. London: HarperCollins.

Ostafin, B D and Kashan, K T (2012) Stepping Out of History: Mindfulness Improves Insight Problem Solving. *Consciousness and Cognition*, 21(2): 1031–6.

Parlerisa, C (2019) Can Mindfulness Actually Help You Work Smarter? *The Keyword*. [online] Available at: https://blog.google/inside-google/life-at-google/mindfulness-at-work (accessed 29 September 2022).

Prabhu, V, Sutton, C and Sauser, W (2008) Creativity and Certain Personality Traits. Understanding the Mediating Effect of Intrinsic Motivation. *Creativity Research Journal*, 20(1): 53–66.

Sandkühler, S and Bhattacharya, J (2008) Deconstructing Insight EEG Correlates of Insight Problem Solving. *PLOS One*, 3(1): 1–12.

Schachtan, N (2013) In Silicon Valley, Meditation Is No Fad. It Could Make Your Career. *Wired*. [online] Available at: www.wired.com/2013/06/meditation-mindfulness-silicon-valley/ (accessed 18 August 2022).

Schooler, J W, Ohlsson, S and Brolls, K (1993) Thoughts Beyond Words: When Language Overshadows Insight. *Journal of Experimental Psychology General*, 122: 166–83.

Sedlmeier, P, Ebeth, J, Schwarz, M, Zimmermann, D, Haarig, F and Jaeger, S (2012) The Psychological Effects of Meditation: A Meta-Analysis. *Psychological Bulletin*, 138(6): 1139–71.

Social Work England (2022) Professional Standards. [online] Available at: www.socialworkengland.org.uk/standards/professional-standards (accessed 28 September 2022).

Chapter 7

Supervision and critical reflection

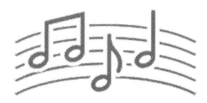

Playing notes or making music?

(Kadushin, 1992)

Supervision has been a longstanding feature of social work, with its earliest presence noted in the 1900s (Kardushin, 1992). While there continues to be uncertainty about the exact contribution supervision makes to the improvement and sustainability of good social work practice (Buckley, 2002), it is generally acknowledged as a good thing. It has been recognised as a necessary forum in which to reflect, evaluate, discuss and develop innovative solutions.

Crucially, in a complex, rapidly changing world, supervision, formal or otherwise, allows for time to stop and reflect, opportunities to weigh the strengths and weaknesses of actions and space to explore feelings engendered by the work.

Mindfulness has a place in social work supervision, as it does in all other aspects of practice. Its presence brings with it the intense learning experience provided in an atmosphere of support and encouragement identified by Munro et al (1989). But above all else, mindfulness is perfectly situated to facilitate the kind of supervision summarised by Davys and Beddoe (2010): '*Supervision can at very best allow, albeit briefly, the doors to be shut, the noise to be reduced and a quiet space for satisfying professional conversation.*'

This chapter will include:

What good looks like

The mindful supervision lens

Intent

Awareness

Critical reflection

Mindful support in supervision

Gratitude

What good looks like

Notwithstanding some of the difficulties in establishing a direct correlation between social work supervision and benefit to service users, supervision has much to offer the social work practitioner. It provides space in which learning, development, critical reflection and personal/professional support can take place. In the absence of the concept of supervision, it is difficult to imagine an alternative mechanism that would provide support to these and any other elements of social work practice.

It is generally accepted that the features of good supervision coalesce around three main functions: education, support and management. This formation can probably be identified within most social work models. It is a triumvirate that provides structure; however, maintaining balance of the three related areas is important. Overemphasis of one aspect at the expense of the others can lead to deficits in the supervision process, an unsatisfactory situation from the perspectives of all who have an investment in the success of supervision.

The four-by-four-by-four model

Acknowledged as one of the most comprehensive concepts of supervision, Wonnacott (2012), in the four-by-four-by-four model, has created a supervision framework that is nested in organisational expectations, but which also references the educational and reflective elements highly regarded within the profession.

The framework identifies four beneficiaries of the supervision process: service users, staff, organisations and partners; four functions of supervision: management, development, support and mediation; and four components of supervision itself: experience, reflection, analysis and planning and action. Wonnacott, along with others such as Munro et al (1989), identifies the activity of reflection as integral to the whole process; without reflection, developmental learning, transitional thinking and problem-solving would not take place. Morrison (2003) highlights the difficulty that can be encountered if all elements of supervision identified by Wonnacott are not implemented in unison, namely inactivity, either as a result of excessive deliberation, loss of focus or fear of action. The model helps to identify the dynamics involved in any supervision activity, creates a point of reference for participants and gives shape to what could easily become a friendly chat that serves little purpose.

Table 7.1 Four by four by four model of supervision

Service users	Developmental	Experience
Staff	Support	Reflection
Organisation	Managerial	Analysis
Partners	Mediation	Plans/actions

While Wonnacott identifies supervision as the thread that holds these elements together in a space that enables an objective lens, it is not always easy to ensure all components receive attention in pursuit of this holistic approach. It has been noted that in recent decades there has tended to be an overemphasis on the managerial or bureaucratic aspects of supervision at the expense of development through reflection or the support needed to meet the emotional demands of the role. The neglect of developmental and emotional features of supervision at the expense of increased attention to bureaucracy can reduce supervision to a perfunctory activity that, while fulfilling the requirements of the organisation at one level, excludes the social work need for supportive development, resulting in staff turnover and poor practice. The difference in the efficacy of supervision in this environment can be that between *playing notes or making music* (Kadushin, 1992).

Take-home message

Education, support and managerial functions are important for supervision that benefits all. However, balance is the key.

Research has also demonstrated that social workers do value supervision, and the supervisory relationship is well regarded. Supervisees emphasise the need for trust in the supervisor/supervisee relationship in order for healthy discussion and collaboration to flow. Further essential qualities identified include positive attitudes, openness and listening (Hughes, 2010).

Supervision enables a review of social work competency, allowing developmental needs to support growth in skill and knowledge. Professional accountability can be maintained, ensuring processes and procedures are followed and gaps in services are identified and considered. In a profession fraught with emotional challenges and stress, supervision provides moments in which to consider well-being. Perhaps one of its most important features is the opportunity it provides to detach from the cycle of reaction to pressure, to critically reflect about the nature of the work, to decide a right course of action and process emotions and feelings engendered by the nature of the work (Davies and Collings, 2008), reflection that allows skillful thought about strengths, risks, needs and safety in relation to cases, enabling smart, creative solutions to problems.

The mindful supervision lens

 Mindfulness can make a significant contribution to the quality of supervision, the supervisory relationship and the homeostatic balance of its features. Traits generated through mindful practice, such as intent, awareness and compassion, have value in their transference to supervision by the mindful social worker, and indeed the mindful supervisor.

Intent

Strong intention is like a rudder to navigate us through the stormy seas
(O'Leary, 2020)

Mindfulness develops awareness of the importance of intention in activity; intention is a present-moment development rather than a future-goal-orientated concept. It gives attention to the purpose of an action and the direction of travel that needs to be held in view. Intent enables fortitude and consistency in the face of difficulty or adversity. In mindfulness meditation, opportunities are taken to check if the right course is being pursued and whether it is necessary to reconstruct or recommit to the original intention. This mindful practice of intention holds many positive possibilities for enhancing the quality of social work supervision.

Developing a shared intention within the social work supervisory relationship secures a strong foundation for the success of supervision in all its features. While it is customary to establish a supervisory agreement that clarifies the purpose of and arrangements for supervision, mindful intention can increase the efficacy of such an agreement, bringing with it a negotiation about the nature of the supervision commitment, the need for both parties to be fully present to the process and the values that should inform discussion. Agreement about intentions serves to help establish trust, honesty and openness, desired characteristics for a good supervisory relationship. Intention provides clarity of action that supports a deeper level of understanding, both between the professionals involved and also of the work under consideration.

Shared intent suggests a collaboration the brings authenticity to supervision, creating an environment that goes some way to fostering the key conditions for good supervision:

- clarity of purpose;

- emotional competence;

- psychological safety;

- accurate assessment of the worker's competencies;

- positive modelling by the supervisor;

- user centredness;

- skill and knowledge enhancement.

(Morrison, 2003)

Mindful point of reflection

Consider what your intentions are in supervision. How do you ensure your commitment to the process? How do you get the best from the supervision opportunities?

Practice example

Table 7.2 Supervision contract

Standard supervision contracting	Mindful supervision intent
Specification of time and dates of supervision	Confirmation of intention
Agreement about responsibilities	Establishment of what each participant will bring to supervision
Agreement about steps taken if supervision missed	Shared acknowledgement of purpose and what is to be achieved.
Understanding of the purpose of supervision	Sharing of values, experiences, skills that each brings to the supervision session
Agreement about how to resolve conflict	Undertaking to commit to attend and honour each others' contributions

Just as O'Leary (2020) uses the metaphor of a rudder employed to navigate stormy seas to illustrate the part intention can play in meditation, so too can a shared intention help one to navigate the successes and pitfalls of the supervision session. Intention acts as a stabilising influence to which both supervisee and supervisor can return if supervision strays off course or participants have lost their way.

Practice example

Arpita has listened to Bernard for some time while he explained how his service user needed help with daily-living tasks but was unwilling to use savings to pay for services. Arpita noticed during this period that she had not heard much of the adult voice in Bernard's presentation of his case. She questioned Bernard, but found he was dismissive of her challenge. Arpita returned to the shared intent of supervision that they had revisited at the beginning of the supervision session. She reminded Bernard of their shared values, in particular person-centred practice. This prompted Bernard to a shift in reflection back to the adult voice, progressing to a more useful discussion about the adult's wishes and strengths and what they might think a 'good life' would be. Bernard was able to surface his own frustrations about the case, including his feelings of helplessness about the provision of services in this instance. Arpita was able to offer support and make space for collaboration about how Bernard might have a strengths-based conversation with his service user that recognised her personal qualities, strengths and support networks and prioritised her outcomes, within which a more holistic plan might be agreed that may or may not involve funding for services.

Shared intention provides a means to mitigate supervision dysfunction occurring through challenging behaviour such as avoidance or stagnation, difficulties that can throw supervision off balance to the detriment of the supervisee and subsequent user services. A return to shared intention, reconnecting (or, as O'Leary (2020) describes it, *'course correcting'*), helps to shift focus beyond the problem towards solutions.

Awareness

 Mindfully sitting still in silence, focusing on the breath and watching thoughts travel past without engagement is a foundational practice of mindfulness and mindful meditation. The observational quality develops the ability to observe both internal and external events in the present, allowing one to notice those things that would normally pass by, fine-tuning perception with the ability to broaden the picture to include all the information that is available beyond a narrowed personal interpretation. This technique has value within the supervision context, extending understanding not only to the events of a case but also to the practitioners' role and the context in which the social work intervention is taking place, leading one to notice requirements of social work practice that can become lost under pressure or through a lack of attendance to present discussion. A mindful approach inspires a 360-degree conversation about the specific details of the service user's issues, but also enables them to be placed in social work interaction and in the context of the wider social justice agenda (Figure 7.1).

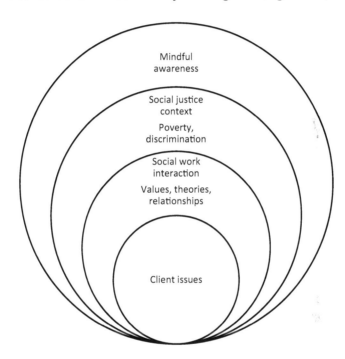

Figure 7.1 Mindfulness awareness in supervision

Practice example

Mindful attention facilitates the placement of child-neglect issues not only within the parenting framework but also within the framework of social work interaction theories, values and research and the wider context of poverty, issues of poor housing, health, education and job prospects.

This in turn adds depth to the understanding of the work under consideration, initiating richer, more-responsive paths of enquiry or response.

Take-home message

Mindful awareness can expand the bandwidth of supervision, adding further depth and understanding to the activity.

Mindfully generated awareness enables greater vigilance over both the content and breadth of supervision discussions, bringing attention to all work that demands scrutiny, as well as to the issues as the supervisee presents them. Such action shines light into the areas of work that can be forgotten or masked by supervision participants' reluctance to discuss them, enabling a comprehensive supervision discussion that considers all work evenly rather than reactively according to the anxiety of either supervisee or supervisor, and engendering awareness that can enable increased focus on preventative actions within social work, recognising lower-level problems that need attention before they escalate into significant events that are only served by often ill-timed or ill-considered emergency decision-making.

Awareness in this fuller sense supports the accurate assessment of the worker's competencies as well as the user-centredness and the supervisor-modelling elements of Morrison's key conditions for good supervision.

Critical reflection

One of the components that distinguishes social work from other helping practices is the essential requirement of critical reflection as part of the role. Supervision provides the opportunity for such reflection, an undertaking that discourages automatic reactionary behaviour in favour of more-considered analytical responses that can provide transformative personal outcomes for service users, with a shift away from habitual response towards present reality.

> *You are just doing task after task and never reflecting on what you are doing... people make assumptions and just race through the work.*
> (Doxtdator, 2012)

The desirable goal of social work that serves the individual necessitates the interruption of repetitive, prescriptive response in favour of something more genuine that relates to the actual circumstances of the person the social worker is seeking to serve; critical thinking turbo-charged with mindfulness can provide the means of achieving this happy state.

Critical thinking, or reflection, is rooted in ancient Greek philosophy, with a belief that the ancient word 'kritikos' refers to the ability to judge (Beyer, 1995). However, the modern model of critical thinking or reflection in use today originates with John Dewey. Dewey (1910) defined reflective thinking as *'active, persistent and careful consideration of any belief or supposed form of knowledge in the light of the grounds that support it'*, emphasising the need to move beyond memorising information for repetition towards the contemplation of information, meaning and application. Critical reflection, within the social work supervisory setting, enables the application of research, evidence and knowledge to decisions and actions in cases. It links experience, skills and knowledge with emotions, thinking and action. Faced with complex human situations, critical reflection can help us to make sense of information, providing insight about the next, most appropriate steps.

Practice example

Murdoch frequently forgets his medication; this has some detrimental effects on his physical health. A response from his social worker is to put in place medication reminders to help Murdoch remember to take his pills. This is an automatic response on the social worker's part, based solely on the observation that Murdoch is 75, his memory might not be as it once was, and this solution has been proven to work in similar situations previously. This may well work and be all that is needed in this case.

However, as time continues and the situation remains the same, with Murdoch being subject to short hospital stays as a result of his not taking medication, some closer critical reflection in supervision is worthwhile. Drawing together of all the information might provide greater insight. The facts include: Murdoch's previous career as a lawyer; his love of

$\longrightarrow$

crosswords; his recent loss of his wife. Analysing his motivation, what would motivate Murdoch to pay closer attention to his medication? Critical reflection yields different areas for exploration with regard to Murdoch, such as what a good life looks like for him, where medication might play a part in that life and what his other strengths or supports are. It transpires that Murdoch is very alert and engaged in numerous activities but finds the medication is dulling his senses and mind, making him confused. This leads to a discussion about the benefits and side effects of medication with his GP, who is able to prescribe different ways of managing pain associated with his current physical condition, minimising his need to use tablets that have negative effects for his cognitive well-being.

The initial, automatic response of the social worker did not meet with success, as the situation involved more than mere memory loss associated with older age. This response may have been appropriate if it matched the personal circumstances of the service user. However, the second response, which encompassed critical reflection on all the information and recognition of Murdoch's strengths, choices and control, led to a change that matched his life goals.

Critical reflection within supervision is an activity that needs to be undertaken carefully and with focus; the consequences of mistakes in such a process may come at a high human cost. Consequently, any aid to the success of critical thinking or reflection is welcome. Mindfulness develops qualities that can offer this positive impact for the success of this activity.

Skobalj (2018) makes a strong case for the benefits of mindfulness in relation to critical thought or reflection within the sphere of education, one that translates easily across professional fields into social work training and practice. Skobalj (2018) recognises attributes of mindfulness beyond its capacity for stress reduction: *'The goal of mindfulness is certainly more far reaching than simply coping with stress and attaining a state of relaxation'.*

Skobalj, like many others, adopts the position that mindfulness enhances certain traits that amplify personal skills of critical thought and reflection. These traits are deemed examples of higher-order brain activity, demanding more complex skills than lower-order repetitive tasks that can be performed as rehearsed or practised automatic responses (for example, eating or running). Critical thought, therefore, requires activation of executive functions of the brain, and these executive areas are believed to respond positively to mindful practice (Chambers et al, 2007; Josefsen and Broberg, 2011; Tang et al, 2012). The mindful components of present-moment attention, alongside non-reactive monitoring of self, serve to enhance clarity of thought, this non-reactive observation supports unbiased analysis of information, reinforced by the mindful skill of emotional self-regulation that limits emotionally driven judgement. Young (1997) also argue that present-moment attention restricts the mind from wandering away from intended goals, reducing ambiguity about the direction of thought. This can be important within social work in order to encourage movement from mere analysis towards enacting the right course of action, tackling the problem of a supervisee or supervisor who is locked in the reflection stage of supervision and unable to move to the next stage of the process. Mindfulness can help to provide the optimum circumstances for critical reflection to take place in a social work supervisory setting by supporting the executive functions of the mind in a way that encourages critical thought, a step up from automatic reactivity or rehearsed practice.

Take-home message

Mindfulness enhances higher-order executive brain functioning, enabling the meditator to step up to the extra challenge of critical thought.

Mindful practice that enables the practitioner to build skill and understanding in sitting with thoughts as they arise translates into the observation not only of external events and people but also of the interior world and how self functions, in particular regarding one's reactions to the surroundings. Such interior knowledge of self strengthens insight into self as a social work practitioner, allowing one to bring to any discussion about practice an understanding of the part that self as a social worker plays in interventions (concerning, for example what values are applied, what judgements are made, and reactions to events that may provoke a compassionate or anxious response). In the context of the internal insight process, self-knowledge also yields responsibility and greater self-regulation, which are necessary characteristics of an insightful, critical conversation about social work in supervision. An acceptance of professional responsibility, alongside regulation, enables the social worker or supervisor to adopt a considered approach to the reflective nature of the work to be discussed, preparing the way for critical thinking. This includes consideration of all the information available, discerning its source, its credibility and whether there are any gaps that need further investigation. It also enables more-detailed thought about the weight and meaning to be attached (or not) to the pieces of information available. The neutral gaze that mindfulness makes available, when deployed in a social work supervision setting, allows us to consider work through a broader lens, bringing into focus the information relating to the service user's issue, the wider context in which the work is enacted and the social worker themselves as representative of a professional intervention.

While there is further exploration needed in relation to mindfulness in this area, studies are beginning to concur with the view that mindfulness can enhance critical thinking, particularly among those who are trained meditation practitioners.

Take-home message

In short, mindful practice facilitates many of the human features of measured, considered and neutral thought and observation. These in turn enable critical thinking to take place in social work, unhindered by obstacles such as personal judgement, procrastination or out-of-control emotions. Mindfulness enables a grown-up supervision conversation.

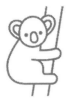

You do not have to hug, but reassurance and support is helpful in social work

Mindful support in supervision

Mindfulness practice engenders compassion for self as well as for others (Shapiro et al, 2005); it teaches the mindful social worker how to recognise feelings, thoughts and emotions and how to regulate them, as well as how to soothe self while containing distress to prevent its escalation to a more serious mental or physical condition (Muscara). There seems to be little to lose and everything to gain by introducing mindfulness into the supervisory arena as a means of accentuating well-being. The mindful social worker, particularly if acting as a supervisor, can be more present to recognise the emotions and feelings of the supervisee undertaking difficult practice. Mindfulness enables both supervision participants to be able to sit together with discomfort, a skill borne out of mindful meditation, and one that is relevant to the difficult material that can come to the fore in a supervision session. This mindful talent of facing uncomfortable or distressing situations opens the gateway to better support and compassion in the supervisory meeting, support that will help others to face their personal or professional challenges on a surer footing.

Munro (2011) identified that social work comes at a high personal cost; with continued exposure to powerful and negative emotions, a lack of effective supervision increases the risk of burnout, emotional exhaustion and cynicism, resulting in reduced personal accomplishment. It is important, therefore, to have the right help and emotional support in supervision, to maintain the balance between all elements of the process, with equal emphasis on well-being alongside managerial expectations. Part of the skillset of a social work supervisor must include kindness, empathy and acceptance alongside the ability to challenge and scrutinise.

Supervision should be a safe environment in which for workers to deal with uncertainty and discuss weaknesses and failings (Englebert, 2014); this condition is necessary for the prevention of the kinds of deterioration referred to by Munro (2011).

The mindful practice of compassion to self enables the mindful supervisor to recognise and be present for the struggles presented by the supervisee, as they learn to listen with patience, empathy, kindness and an understanding that can soothe conflictual emotions and feelings in supervision, enabling the supervisee to attempt recovery of self and self-preservation to prevent emotional burnout. 'When emotional support *is provided well in supervision there are lower levels of negative outcomes associated with stress'* (Lloyd et al, 2002).

Practice example

A supervisee confides in supervision that they are struggling with a case; they are trying their best but failing to make connections, and they have become concerned that they have tried all the actions they can think of but may have missed something. A child has been injured during a spontaneous domestic violence incident; initial independent enquiries have concluded that the incident could not have been foreseen based on the information available to social services.

While there will be a time for them later, it would be unhelpful to apply process or accountability discussions as an opening to this conversation. A compassionate, supportive approach, which can be developed during mindful practice, would be to listen empathetically, acknowledge the supervisee's feelings about the case and provide comfort and reassurance, thus enabling a gentle move towards discussion of the events and the strengths of the supervisee's intervention, while also identifying areas for knowledge and skill development.

Mindfulness practice encourages the essential quality of compassion as the practitioner sits watching thoughts arise, whatever they are, without judgement, simultaneously teaching kindness to and forgiveness of self. In a world where it becomes impossible to meet the exacting standards we set for ourselves, to compete in what is perceived on social media as a high-achieving society, and with the growth of continual self-disapproval due to lack of success in comparison, compassion for self as well as others provides a central rock to help stem the ever-rising tide of self-criticism. The use of compassion within the social work supervisory relationship is an act capable of enabling equanimity in the face of the pressures of the social work role, helping to contain the most extreme of emotions that can be triggered by working with humanity in all its manifestations. *'One of the major functions of supervision involves containing or managing anxiety and helping to cope with the demands that the work entails'* (Brearley, 1995).

There can be no doubt that compassion can add considerably to one's ability to manage anxiety, helping one to come to terms with the demands of social work described by Brearley (1995). Compassion is an inherent characteristic that is deemed to be present within everyone. It cannot be taught, but needs to be given attention in order to fully develop. Mindful practice that allows thoughts to arise without judgement, without expectation, and to be treated with kindness, facilitates the development of this trait. Greater mindful practice brings with it increased competency, translating compassion for self into the social work supervisory relationship. Compassion allows vulnerability and uncertainty to be present; everything can be unpacked – feelings, emotions, information, questions – forming the basis of open, honest supervision discussion in a safe space, that can lead to transformative practice both for the individuals and those they support. Giving mindful attention to compassion in supervision translates into mindful compassionate social work practice, enabling the practitioner to be better present for the vulnerabilities and uncertainties expressed by service users, promoting conversations about support that are more insightful and with the potential for wiser, more collaborative proportionate, responsive interventions.

Gratitude

I can live for two months on a good compliment.

(Mark Twain)

 Mindful cultivation of gratitude also has a positive part to play in social work supervision. Mindful attention to the things that make us thankful correlates with many of the social work models of strengths-based practice that promote attention to that which is going well rather than only that which is problematic – noticing the light as well as the dark in any given situation. Mindfulness teaches awareness of all things and to have gratitude for what is going well in our lives. It also teachers us to have gratitude for the good fortune of others. This practice in turn helps to develop generosity of spirit together with an understanding of the transient nature of things, helping us recognise the importance of being thankful for whatever there is. Many mindful practitioners focus on gratitude as part of meditation or keep a daily log or diary of things in the day

to be thankful for. This habit reinforces the more positive aspects of our nature: while we are thankful for what we have ourselves, the practice generates gratitude in the workplace and can become a feature of supervision that balances or motivates the supervisee.

In recent times, the power of being thankful has been evident in the commitment to applaud the NHS for their extraordinary work during the Covid-19 pandemic, an activity that demonstrates the power of thankfulness to sustain healthcare professionals under extreme pressure and bind neighbourhoods and communities in a shared positive action during a bleak time. Such a characteristic is equally able to support social workers in a supervisory relationship by enabling the supervisor to notice opportunities to thank the supervisee for their work or participation in supervision. A small act, thanking someone for actions or work that might otherwise go unnoticed builds a person's confidence and self-esteem, demonstrating to them that they are a valued employee.

Several studies have examined the effect that thoughtfulness or gratitude can have on staff. One of them, a recent study between Kings College London and Harvard Business school, concentrated on the effect gratitude can have on the social work profession in particular. The study divided social workers randomly into two groups: members of one group received a letter of thanks for their work from their line manager; the other group received nothing. Several months later, the recipients of the letter of thanks confirmed they felt more valued than their counterparts who had no such communication of gratitude (Bartleby, 2022), demonstrating the power of gratitude and how it translates into changes in the quality of the social work workplace. Similarly, a study involving employees of Coca-Cola secretly requested that some of the workers carry out acts of kindness towards a smaller group of colleagues. Both the givers and the recipients of these acts reported higher levels of job satisfaction, and receivers ended up passing on acts of kindness to others (Bartleby, 2022). Two features of mindfulness, gratitude and small acts of kindness, are able to have transformative effects on employees and the workplace. The presence of these two actions within a supervision session has the power to enhance well-being and the kindness of the social work environment, changes that will benefit social workers and colleagues, and by extension those who access services.

Take-home message

Remembering to add gratitude and kindness into supervision and the rest of the day can be a small act with big positive impact. Supervision can be used as a launch point from which to change the social work mood.

 Mindfulness, woven like a thread through supervision, influences several of the key ingredients that Morrison (2003) thinks make for good supervision. Above all, it serves to create a safe space for a good conversation, a place where the supervisee and supervisor can place trust in each other without laying blame. Feelings and actions can be explored during time spent away from the everyday management or crisis-driven practice that dogs social work. Each participant can emerge with renewed perspectives and motivation and the confidence to continue with the demands of the job, whether as supervisor or supervisee. The alchemy of mindfulness supports a refresh or reset during supervision, making it the perfect travel companion for supervisory progress.

 # Takeaways

1. Key points

- Supervision is the only viable, recognised mechanism through which educational, managerial and supportive functions can combine to support the social worker in practice.

- Social workers report that they value supervision and find it helpful, if only for the space and time it allows for reflection about work and the processing of the myriad feelings and emotions that the work engenders.

- Mindfulness can support high-quality supervision by establishing intent, a feature that both supervisor and supervisee navigate by when things become difficult.

- Mindfulness can expand the bandwidth of supervision, adding greater depth and understanding.

$\longrightarrow$

- Executive functioning is enhanced through mindful practice. Functioning at this level is needed for critical reflection about social work practice in supervision.

- Mindful inclusion of kindness, gratitude and compassion in a supervision session translates not only into improved relationships between participants but also into benefits for the wider social work field.

2. Topics for mindful supervision

Intention and commitment ⟶ What will that look like?

Getting the balance right ⟶ Are all three elements present in each supervision?

Critical reflection ⟶ How will we notice when it is time to move from analysis to the next stage of critical reflection?

Points of gratitude ⟶ Where can thanks be given?

Small acts of kindness ⟶ Identify where kindness can be offered.

Checking well-being ⟶ Note the importance of support and quiet space for a good conversation.

3. Support pillars for mindful supervision

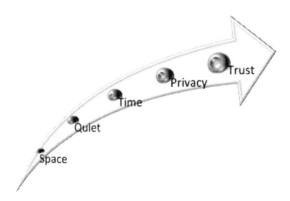

Figure 7.2 Support pillars for mindful supervision

References and further reading

Bartleby (2022) The Power of Small Gestures, Showing Appreciation Is an Art Not a Science. *The Economist*, 28 May.

Beyer, B K (2017) *Critical Thinking.* Bloomington: Phi Delta Kappa Educational Foundation.

Brearley, J (1995) *Counselling and Social Work*. Buckingham: Open University Press.

Buckley, H (2008) *Child Protection Work: Beyond the Rhetoric*. London: Jessica Kingsley.

Chambers, R, Lo, B C and Allen, N B (2007) The Impact of Intensive Mindfulness Training on Attentional Control, Cognitive Style and Affect. *Cognitive Therapy and Research*, 32(3): 303–22.

Colzato, L S, Ozturk, A and Hommel, B (2012) Meditate to Create: The Impact of Focused-Attention and Open-Monitoring Training on Convergent and Divergent Thinking. *Frontiers in Psychology*, 3: 116.

Davys, A and Beddoe, L (2020) *Best Practice in Professional Supervision*, 2nd edition. London: Jessica Kingsley.

Davies, L and Collings, S (2008) Emotional Knowledge for Child Welfare Practice: Rediscovering Our Roots. *Smith College Studies in Social Work*, 78(1): 7–26.

Dewey, J (1910) *How We Think*. Chicago: D C Heath and Co Publishers.

Doxtdator (2012) *Mindfulness: Helping Social Workers Bring Themselves Home*. Ontario: McMaster University.

Engelbrecht, L (2014) Social Work Supervision Policies and Frameworks: Playing Notes or Making Music? *Social Work*, 49(4): 456–68.

Fook, J (1996) *The Reflective Researcher: Social Workers' Theories of Practice Research*. Sydney: Allen and Unwin.

Hughes, J M (2010) The Role of Supervision in Social Work: A Critical Analysis. *Critical Social Thinking: Policy and Practice*, 2. [online] Available at: www.ucc.ie/en/media/academic/appliedsocialstudies/docs/JeanneHughes.pdf (accessed 18 August 2022).

Jackson, K (2020) The Mindful Social Worker: How Mindfulness Can Help Social Workers Practice More Creatively. *Social Work Today*, 17(5): 14.

Josefsson, T and Broberg, A (2011) Meditators and Non-Meditators on Sustained and Executive Attentional Performance. *Mental Health, Religion and Culture*, 14: 291–309.

Kadushin, A (1992) *Supervision in Social Work.* New York: Columbia University Press.

Kettle, M (2015) Achieving Effective Supervision. [online] Available at: www.iriss.org.uk/resources/insights/achieving-effective-supervision (accessed 18 August 2022).

Lloyd, C, King, R and Chenoweth, L (2002) Social Work, Stress and Burnout: A Review. *Journal of Mental Health*, 11(3): 255–65.

Morrison, T (2003) *Staff Supervision in Social Care.* Southampton: Ashford Press.

Munro, A, Manthei, B and Small, J (1989) *Counselling: The Skills of Problem Solving.* London: Routledge.

Munro, E (2011) *The Munro Review of Child Protection: Final Report – A Child-Centred System.* London: Department for Education.

Noone, C, Buntin, B and Hogan, M (2015) Does Mindfulness Enhance Critical Thinking? Evidence for the Mediating Effects of Executive Functioning in the Relationship between Mindfulness and Critical Thinking. *Frontiers in Psychology*, 6: 2043.

O'Leary, W (2020) A 4-Step Practice to Awaken your Intention. *Mindful.org*. [online] Available at: www.mindful.org/4-ways-to-awaken-your-intention/ (accessed 20 September 2022).

Ostafin, B D and Kashan, K T (2012) Stepping out of History: Mindfulness Improves Insight Problem Solving. *Consciousness and Cognition*, 21(2): 1031–6.

Parlerisa, C (2019) Mindfulness at Work. [online] Available at: https://blog.google/inside-google/life-at-google/mindfulness-at-work (accessed 18 August 2022).

Schachtan, N (2013) In Silicon Valley, Meditation Is No Fad. It Could Make Your Career. *Wired*, 18 June. [online] Available at: www.wired.com/2013/06/meditation-mindfulness-silicon-valley/ (accessed 18 August 2022).

Shapiro, S L, Astin, J A, Bishop, S R and Cordova, M (2005) Mindfulness-based Stress Reduction for Health Care Professionals: Results from a Randomized Trial. *International Journal of Stress Management*, 12: 164–76.

Skobalj, E (2018) Mindfulness and Critical Thinking: Why Should Mindfulness Be the Foundation of the Educational Process? *University Journal of Educational Research*, 37(6): 1365–72.

Tang, Y-Y, Yang, L, Leve, D L and Harold, G T (2012) Improving Executive Function and Its Neurobiological Mechanisms through a Mindfulness Intervention, Advances within the Field of Developmental Neuroscience. *Child Development Perspectives*, 6: 316–66.

Wonnacott, J (2012) *Mastering Social Work Supervision*. London: Jessica Kingsley.

Young, S (1997) *The Science of Enlightenment*. Boulder, CO: Sounds True.

Chapter 8

Conclusion: continuing the mindful journey

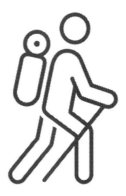

I am getting something out of this, so I am going to stick with it
(Masheder et al, 2020)

Academic research and conversation indicate that mindfulness is showing all the signs of becoming a very useful adjunctive tool that not only builds resilience and well-being within the social work professional but also transforms practice to the benefit of service user groups, a shift very much in line with the ultimate goal of social work, which is a practice that seeks to serve people well. Presence in the moment creates a movement of focus away from past and future events, which result in an unhelpful cycle of an unbalanced awareness of risk leading to catastrophic thinking, creating space for a more balanced development of interpersonal skills alongside evidence-based assessment and decision-making, while also enhancing the practitioner's ability to find the creative solutions required to meet individual circumstances.

However, because of the personal nature of mindful practice, it is inevitable that change begins with the individual journey of the social worker to explore the possibilities of mindful practice for themselves. Once the decision to become a mindful social worker is made, developing, and sustaining the mindful approach can prove challenging in the face of daily stress and competing demands on time. This chapter provides further reading and resources to support social workers who are interested in beginning the journey, alongside the Resource hut, which is intended to help the practitioner continue to navigate a mindful professional path, mitigating the effects of stress and work pressures that might threaten to undo progress. Continued development of mindful practice yields greater benefits, and the resources in this chapter are intended to sow the seeds for a mindful social work career.

This chapter will include:

To 'stop and drop'

Not just another thing

Relaxing into mindfulness

Best endeavour

Rewards

Overcoming resistance

Getting by with a little help from some friends

At this point in the mindful social work exploration, the benefits of mindfulness both for self and for practice are evident in regard to social work; a summary is provided in the 'Takeaways' section as a reminder and to address any doubt. But the challenge to come is the adoption of a continued mindful practice that can be sustained for life. One of the joys of mindfulness is that it is a unique practice for each individual. Its quality of non-striving is a welcome antidote to the often ferocious world of competitive performance in all that we do. Mindfulness is personal; it evolves in a way that defines the character and nature of each individual's practice, and in that way it becomes a very special, private space. The journey involves finding out about self, how self-mind works, and being able to manage self in action, whether in a personal or social work setting, ultimately leading to positive changes that bring to the fore inner peace, kindness, compassion, gratitude and wise action, allowing the practitioner to see the light as well as the dark in all things, because this provides balance for well-being.

To 'stop and drop'

Mindfulness is experiential, it is a state of being that involves tuning into the ability to notice the mind: 'stop and drop' (a phrased coined by Kabat-Zinn) into the present moment. Talking about the subject may be helpful for establishing support or shared experience, but too much talking can have the effect of draining the experience of mindfulness, and Kabat-Zinn warns of the dangers of too much mindful conversation. The real power of mindfulness is less about defining self by talking to others about it, and lies more in the experience of being mindful. *'You have to actually practice mindfulness in order to reap it's benefits and come to understand why it is so valuable'* (Kabat-Zinn, 1990). This does not preclude drawing support from undertaking mindfulness practice with others as a shared experience, but talking about it transfers the depth of experience from self to increased chatter in the mind, which inhibits the development of insight and growth of personhood.

Not just another thing

Consideration of personal commitment is also of value when seeking to embed mindfulness in life. It is important that mindfulness, particularly formal meditation mindfulness, does not just become another thing to do, a further burden within a busy life. Perhaps the most desirable context would be one wherein mindfulness becomes integral to all that we do, in which meditation is as routine as brushing our teeth, eating or sleeping. Realisation of this arrangement can only take place when we review and adjust the life structure we use to help us live in the short and long term.

Relaxing into mindfulness

Traditionally, life is lived with goals or aspirations that we strive to achieve, seeking opportunities to develop or enhance skills, knowledge and experiences. These form the bedrock of how we live our lives, the life fabric that is referenced in all that we do. Often, we find ourselves immersed in a pressured living environment that necessitates multi-tasking, plans and prioritisation to enable choices to be made as we seek to gain some control over ever-competing demands. This way of living can be very fruitful, providing senses of achievement and success and the creation of the kind of lifestyle that some would like to live. However, if expectations are too high, often due to our comparison with others or media imaging, a sense of failure or increased self-criticism can occur within our minds, sometimes becoming the dominant message to the exclusion of all that is well. If unchecked, this may become a source of sadness or anxiety, disappointment or loss of self-esteem; it can lead to the abandonment of efforts that could lead to positive change.

A tilt of the life perspective towards the principles of mindfulness is more likely to lead to a sustained, long-term, beneficial practice. In the first instance this means letting go of striving and adopting a more accepting approach that sees mindfulness as a journey of exploration that must be allowed to unfold and not be directed by our desire to achieve. This can come as a welcome relief from the high-achieving, expectant nature of the world. Letting go is the means of living with kindness and compassion to self when things go wrong or when there is no time to practise meditation and it will need to resume at another point. *'Knowing I can always begin again which is very kindly and forgiving'* (Birtwell et al, 2019). Discarding expectations of results or goals in mindfulness can provide the comforting reassurance that should we step off the mindful path, there is no need to worry or admonish self for failure but just to understand that it will always be there when we are ready to take it up again.

Best endeavour

 Setting aside the pursuit of goals, it is a widely accepted truth that mindfulness will not take place without the motivation of the practitioner; it does, therefore, require a desire to practice mindful meditation, or to stop and drop in the moment regularly, in order to be of benefit. Perhaps it is the commitment or intention of the practitioner to pursue mindfulness as an act of self-care that deserves attention; an intention to continue a mindful practice is a sustaining element of that practice, and making best endeavours to maintain practice in a way that is kind to self provides a mindful frame of approach that is likely to yield success.

This will clearly take determination and resolve to aid the journey, but experiencing the benefits during the travel will help to encourage continuation. Making best endeavours includes consideration of how to continue the journey. Spending as little as ten minutes in meditation can have a positive effect on well-being and produce the kinds of benefits highlighted in this book. Planning a ten-minute pause in the day with a little privacy and quiet may mean arriving in the car to work or an appointment early for a peaceful moment, departing later or finding a pause in the middle of the day. If formal meditation is out of the question, adopting a mindful approach to daily tasks will also help positive progress. Something as simple as mindfully eating a piece of fruit at lunchtime can make for a silent pause. What's important is the incorporation of mindfulness into routine within life. This takes an explicit manifestation of intention, with a return when there is an absence of practice, and precludes judging self as a failure or despairing over a loss of ability; just remember your intention and return to the activity; it will always be there as an innate quality throughout life.

Take-home message

Plans are great if they work for you, but remembering to let go of striving and to accept what happens without judgement and with kindness to self are important steps towards sustaining a continued mindful practice.

Rewards

 Identified as one of the most important motivators, reaping the benefits of mindfulness in life has a significant impact on the continuation of practice. As we see benefits manifest in our personal and professional life, the maintenance of practice becomes easier. But this action requires a complete circle (Figure 8.1).

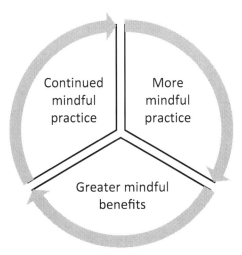

Figure 8.1 Mindfulness reward cycle

The more we practice, the greater the rewards, which in turn motivates us to practice more – a perfect virtuous circle. However, one of the keys to this cycle, is being open to noticing the benefits as they arise. This awareness helps to encourage further mindful practice. One of the helpful ways this can be achieved is through keeping a mindful diary or journal to encourage reflection about self at the beginning of the mindful journey and to record the changes noticed. This has the added benefit of trans-lating more broadly into professional social work life, as you will notice the strengths or positive changes in people receiving social work services over time, charting a visual picture of progress as well as providing a much more balanced approach to personal and professional life.

Once more, this becomes an exercise in managing expectations and accepting what happens. Mindfulness is not having a conversation with fellow practitioners about their benefits and expecting the same will occur for you in the short term. It is a revealing adventure, involving being open to noticing small changes. Even if the only change you find in meditation practice is that you fall asleep, this can be viewed with acceptance as a beneficial, relaxing experience, while you can also take steps to review how to remain wakeful in meditation, perhaps by altering the time of practice. In a study completed by Birtwell et al (2019), participants who fell asleep during meditation still found positives in their experience, highlighting it as a help with insomnia or finding themselves in a more rested, peaceful state on waking than if they had just grabbed a nap.

Overcoming resistance

Finally, we are all human, and part of the journey involves meeting and overcoming resistance. Usually, resistance in mindfulness mirrors our actions of resistance in our daily lives. Sometimes it may take the form of self-sabotage, as when we find successful benefits but are fearful of continuing, or it can take the form of reluctance to continue practice because of anxiety of failure or because it brings to the surface areas that are too difficult to contemplate, reflecting avoidant behaviour.

This poses challenges with regard to fulfilling the intention to be mindful. It requires awareness of what is taking place and determination to continue, but also consideration of adjustments that might need to be made to practice. The adjustments might mean drawing from a support network or seeking professional guidance in meditation or in response to any wider health needs for mental and physical well-being.

The main point is that the process requires recognising what is happening and taking steps to continue even if includes a pause or change to the way mindfulness is practised. Recognising and overcoming resistance from self to make positive change is a valuable human trait that mindfulness can enhance. It translates into social work practice for the mindful social worker, with off-cushion benefits like helping you to identify when there is innate personal/professional resistance to a visit or case, or by providing increased awareness of emotions that can guide adjustments to help overcome any challenge. Inevitably, over time, resilience and tenacity will ensue to build a determined, aware character that can be beneficial to both personal and professional life.

Mindful point of reflection

Consider where your points of resistance lie. How do you avoid doing things that you do not like? What might help you to overcome them? Identifying resistance will help you to navigate it when you encounter it in your mindful practice.

Getting by with a little help from some friends

Most mindfulness participants highlight support from friends, family or a mindful community as the greatest support to maintaining their practice. This can be particularly relevant when being mindful includes being present with difficult emotions or information as well as with positive ones. Whether the people we draw support from are met in person or online makes little difference to motivation; practitioners enjoy the freedom in this technological age to choosing the support that suits self, with the greater being opened up by virtual contact compensating in those areas where direct in-person support is not available.

This need for wider support for mindful living is as salient for those who have dedicated their lives to mindfulness as it is for those new to the experience. In 1966 Buddhist monk and global spiritual leader Thich Nhat Hanh founded a Buddhist order in Plum Village, France, following his departure from Vietnam, his clear intention being to establish a community of likeminded, mindful practitioners that could share their experience, offering support to each other. Indeed, ancient Buddhist teachings reinforce the importance of companionship in practice. Here he is expressing the importance of support with reference to *sangha*, which means 'community':

> *The presence of those who practice mindful living is a great support and encouragement to us... getting in touch with an existing sangha or setting up a small sangha amount to a very important step.*
>
> (Nhat Hanh, 1997)

Newcomers place equal importance on wider mindful support, viewing the opportunity to buddy with friends or groups as a significant motivating factor. Something as simple as texting each other as a reminder to meditate, be mindful or to share a mindful meditation practice sometimes makes the difference between practicing or not.

> *I buddy up with a friend and we text each other when we have completed a formal practice. I taught her mindfulness and now offer informal supervision. This monthly connection keeps me on track.*
>
> (Birtwell et al, 2019)

Motivating support can extend beyond the informal social network to the workplace, as more organisations are recognising the benefits of mindfulness and embracing the practice. The same can be true for social work, with a leading example provided by the State of Victoria, Australia (Australian Association of Social Workers, 2022). Here, social work incorporates a practice of social work combined with yoga and mindfulness that provides opportunities to meet and discuss the topic, as well as providing resources and research. A link to the site is offered in the Resource hut. It provides a lighthouse example of just how encouraging a work culture of mindfulness can be for social work, with early recognition of its value in the workplace.

Take-home message

It may be that as a self-starter you are able to maintain your own personal practice, but companionable support drawn from a place that you identify can make the difference between good practice and an outstanding mindful journey with layers of depth through shared experience.

Takeaways

1. Key points

- One of the pleasures of mindfulness is that it is a personal journey of exploration that includes letting go of striving.

- Remembering to stop and drop into the present is key.

- Best endeavours are all that is required to continued mindfulness, but be aware that should practice be interrupted, it will always be there to resume when you are ready.

- Help from family and friends is great, but talking too much about the practice can take away its power. There is a great deal to be gained from the silent connection of like minds in a mindful way.

- Don't forget to notice the benefits both on- and off-cushion.

2. Suggestions for mindful moments in the day

Upon waking, before getting up

In the shower, noticing the luxury of water

Eating breakfast

Walking to work

On the train journey

Moments in the car dropping children at school or departing from school (it's good to engage the children as well at moments, just to regroup and calm before getting out the car)

Washing up

Brushing teeth

Listening to music

Or just immersing yourself in a good cup of tea

3. 'Reasons to be cheerful, 1, 2, 3!'

Take time at a point in the day to notice and even record three things for which you are grateful, resetting the balance of your day.

4. The summary table of mindful good news for social work

Social work	Mindful enhancement
Well-being	Mindfulness mitigates the negative effects of social work practice, such as stress, burnout and compassion fatigue. Mindfulness produces a calmer state that supports resilience
Communication	Mindfulness changes the brain in ways that enhance the ability to communicate and connect with people. It facilitates increased attention, free from distraction, which adds to awareness of what is truly happening in the moment.

→

Social work	Mindful enhancement
Trusted relationships	Mindfulness promotes qualities that encourage those who are served to place their trust in the social worker: integrity, benevolence and competence.
Assessment	Mindfulness establishes authentic collaboration, creating a shift from habitual reactivity to full awareness, including awareness of self as an agent in social work practice.
Creativity	Mindfulness can unlock our creative nature, allowing it to grow in all that we do. It can lead to increased flexibility and adaptability and make us more agile or responsive in our social work practice.
Supervision	Mindfulness can expand the bandwidth of supervision, adding greater depth and understanding. It can also increase the powers of critical reflection, while bringing gratitude and compassion into activity that is both worthwhile for those involved and to the ultimate benefit of those who are served by social work.

References and further reading

Australian Association of Social Workers (2022) Social Work Yoga and Mindfulness Practice Group. [online] Available at: www.aasw.asn.au/victoria/yoga-and-mindfulness/social-work-yoga-and-mindfulness-practice-group (accessed 28 September 2022).

Birtwell, K, Williams, K, Marwijk, H, Armitage, C and Sheffield, D (2019) An Exploration of Formal and Informal Mindfulness Practice and Associations with Wellbeing. *Mindfulness*, 10(1): 89–99.

Hanley, A W, Waner, A R, Dehili, V M, Canto, A I, and Garland, E L (2015) Washing Dishes to Wash the Dishes: Brief Instruction in an Informal Mindfulness Practice. *Mindfulness*, 6: 1095–103.

Kabat-Zinn, J (1990) *Full Catastrophe Living*. New York: Random House

Kabat-Zinn, J (2011) Foreword. In Williams, M and Penman, D (eds) *Mindfulness: A Practical Guide to Finding Peace in a Frantic World*. London: Piatkus.

Masheder, J, Fjorback, L and Parsons, E (2020) 'I Am Getting Something out of This, so I Am Going to Stick with It': Supporting Participants' Home Practice in Mindfulness-Based Programmes. *BMC Psychology* 8(91). doi. org/10.1186/s40359-020-00453-x.

McCown, D, Reibel, D and Micozzi, M S (2010) *Teaching Mindfulness: A Practical Guide for Clinicians and Educators*. New York: Springer.

Nhat Hahn, T N (1997) *Transformation and Healing: Sutra on the Four Foundations of Mindfulness*. Berkeley: Parallax Press.

Sucitto, A (1988) *Introduction to Insight Meditation*. Hemel Hempstead: Amaravati Publications.

Sucitto, A (2012) Parami: Ways to Cross Life's Floods. Hemel Hempstead: Amaravati Publications.

Sumedho, A (1996) The Mind and the Way: Buddhist Reflections on Life. London: Rider & Co.

Vettese, L C, Toneatto, T, Stea, J N, Nguyen, L and Wang, J (2009) Do Mindfulness Meditation Participants Do Their Homework? And Does It Make a Difference? A Review of the Empirical Evidence. *Journal of Cognitive Psychotherapy: an International Quarterly*, 23(3): 198–225.

Wahbeh, H, Svalina, M N, and Oken, B S (2014) Group, One-on-One, or Internet? Preferences for Mindfulness Meditation Delivery Format and Their Predictors. *Open Medicine Journal*, 1: 66–74.

Williams, M and Penman, D (2011) *Mindfulness: An Eight-Week Plan for Finding Peace in a Frantic World*. Emmaus, PA: Rodale Books.

Resource hut: a place of mindfully good things

A list of places to enjoy mindful smiling moments:

www.royalacademy.org.uk/article/9-virtual-exhibition-art-tours-to-watch-online

www.birminghammuseums.org.uk/bmag/virtual-tour

https://travel.earth//breathtaking-virtual-tours-of-natural-sites/

www.nga.gov/features/true-to-nature-virtual-tour.html

https://virtualnature.com

www.nationaltrust.org.uk//lists/virtual-tours-of-our-places

www.nhm.ac.uk/visit/exhibitions/nature-live.html

https://lightsoverlapland.com//abisko-national-park-virtual-reality-tour/

https://armchair-travels.com//a-virtual-english-seaside-trip/

Mindful meditation places to start

www.smilingmind.com.au//mindfulness/

www.headspace.com/mindfulness

www.headspace.com

https://plumvillage.org//#filter=.region-eu

https://plumvillage.org//live-events/walking-meditation/

Mindful tools to get you started:

Sample templates for your journal

The start of my mindful journey... Fill in the notes below and keep them to remember the good things about life	
	Why it is good to be me
	This is what clouds my days (do less of this!)
	This is what brings me sunshine (do more of this!)
	My first mindful steps will be

Gratitude journal page	
Day:	Date:

There are only two ways to live your life: One is as though nothing is a miracle. The other is as though everything is miracle. (Albert Einstein)

Three things that went well in the day

Three act of kindness today

Three things to be thankful for

Mindful mind map templates

Use the first template to help you populate the second mindful mind map for yourself.

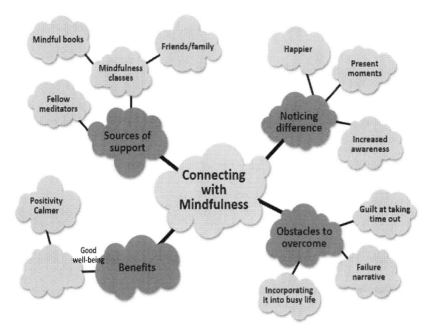

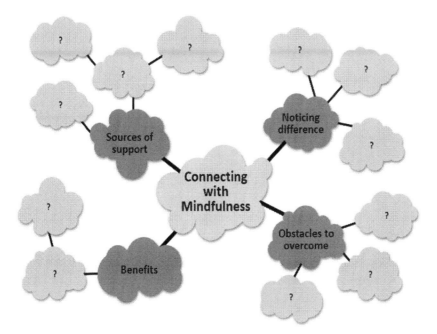

Mindful desk-swipe template

Use this template to remind you to be mindful at work.

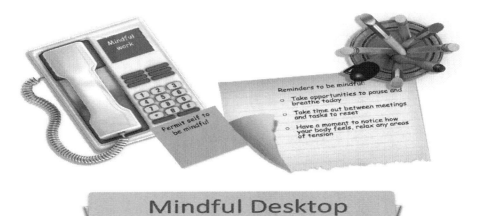

Mindful meditations to get you started

Meditation on compassion

- *Sitting or lying down in a comfortable position, close your eyes and take three long breaths, breathing in through the nose and out through the mouth. As you breathe deeply out, feel yourself letting go of any tension in your body.*

- *Gently return your breath to normal, breathing in and out through your nose. Bring your attention to the breath as it enters and leaves your body. As you breathe in, feel the air entering your body, and as you breathe out, let go of your feelings and thoughts.*

- *Stay with your breath, and without opening your eyes bring your attention to the centre of your chest, the heart centre. Remain with relaxed presence in this area of your body. Notice any feelings of warmth or happiness when you stay in this place for a while.*

- *As your thoughts pass by through the mind, notice any that are negative or self-critical when they arise. Resist engaging in judgement of these thoughts but return attention to the heart centre, bringing to the fore feelings of kindness to self.*

- *Eventually, as thoughts subside, bring to mind an image of the people or places that make you happy. Hold them in place while you feel any warmth or peace at your heart centre. Rest for a time in this space.*

- *When you are ready to return from your meditation, begin to wiggle your toes and fingers to awake. Bring a smile to your face before opening your eyes.*

- *Take a moment to notice how you feel before moving back into present living.*

Relaxing body-scan meditation

- *Sitting or lying down in a comfortable position, close your eyes and take three long breaths, breathing in through the nose and out through the mouth. As you breathe deeply out, feel yourself letting go of any tension in your body.*

- *Gently return your breath to normal, breathing in and out through your nose. Bring your attention to the breath as it enters and leaves your body. As you breathe in, feel the air entering your body, and as you breathe out, let go of your feelings and thoughts.*

- *Without opening your eyes, bring attention to parts of the body starting from the top of the head. You need do nothing other than rest awareness in each part as you move through.*

- *Start with the top of the head, moving down to the forehead, through the face to the jawline and lower to the neck.*

- *Gently rest a while in the shoulder area before moving down each arm to the hands and fingers. Return to the chest and move through the torso to the waist and along each leg to the feet and toes.*

- *Move around the toes and up the back of the body, resting at each stage along the back, arms and neck and at the back of head, and return to the forehead.*

- *Stay here, noticing the breath as it rises and falls within the body.*

- *When you are ready to awaken, simply wiggle your toes and fingers to bring back physical sensation before opening the eyes.*

- *Before moving into your day, notice how relaxed your body feels; this will help you notice tension when it occurs.*

- *This meditation is great for any part of the day, or even at bedtime for a relaxing sleep*

Now is the time to put this book down and ease into mindful social work practice!

Index

Note: Page numbers in **bold** and *italics* denote tables and figures, respectively.